FREE Study Skills Videos/DVD Offer

Dear Customer,

Thank you for your purchase from Mometrix! We consider it an honor and a privilege that you have purchased our product and we want to ensure your satisfaction.

As a way of showing our appreciation and to help us better serve you, we have developed Study Skills Videos that we would like to give you for <u>FREE</u>. These videos cover our *best practices* for getting ready for your exam, from how to use our study materials to how to best prepare for the day of the test.

All that we ask is that you email us with feedback that would describe your experience so far with our product. Good, bad, or indifferent, we want to know what you think!

To get your FREE Study Skills Videos, you can use the **QR code** below, or send us an **email** at studyvideos@mometrix.com with *FREE VIDEOS* in the subject line and the following information in the body of the email:

- The name of the product you purchased.
- Your product rating on a scale of 1-5, with 5 being the highest rating.
- Your feedback. It can be long, short, or anything in between. We just want to know your impressions and experience so far with our product. (Good feedback might include how our study material met your needs and ways we might be able to make it even better. You could highlight features that you found helpful or features that you think we should add.)

If you have any questions or concerns, please don't hesitate to contact me directly.

Thanks again!

Sincerely,

Jay Willis
Vice President
jay.willis@mometrix.com
1-800-673-8175

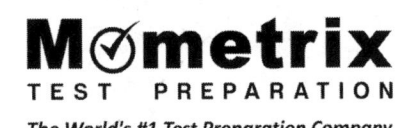

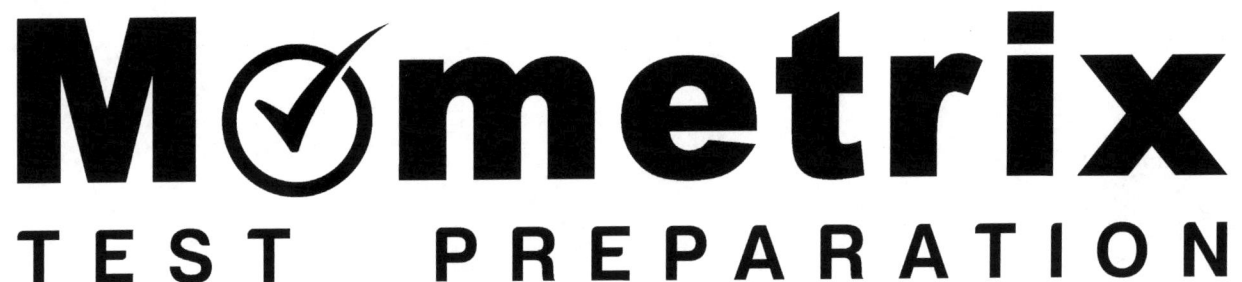

Certified Dialysis Nurse Exam Secrets Study Guide

CDN Test Review for the
Certified Dialysis Nurse Exam

Copyright © 2021 by Mometrix Media LLC

All rights reserved. This product, or parts thereof, may not be reproduced, stored in a retrieval system, or transmitted in any form or by any means—electronic, mechanical, photocopy, recording, scanning, or other—except for brief quotations in critical reviews or articles, without the prior written permission of the publisher.

Written and edited by Mometrix Test Prep

Printed in the United States of America

This paper meets the requirements of ANSI/NISO Z39.48-1992 (Permanence of Paper).

Mometrix offers volume discount pricing to institutions. For more information or a price quote, please contact our sales department at sales@mometrix.com or 888-248-1219.

Mometrix Media LLC is not affiliated with or endorsed by any official testing organization. All organizational and test names are trademarks of their respective owners.

Paperback
ISBN 13: 978-1-60971-297-6
ISBN 10: 1-6097-1297-8

Dear Future Exam Success Story

First of all, **THANK YOU** for purchasing Mometrix study materials!

Second, congratulations! You are one of the few determined test-takers who are committed to doing whatever it takes to excel on your exam. **You have come to the right place.** We developed these study materials with one goal in mind: to deliver you the information you need in a format that's concise and easy to use.

In addition to optimizing your guide for the content of the test, we've outlined our recommended steps for breaking down the preparation process into small, attainable goals so you can make sure you stay on track.

We've also analyzed the entire test-taking process, identifying the most common pitfalls and showing how you can overcome them and be ready for any curveball the test throws you.

Standardized testing is one of the biggest obstacles on your road to success, which only increases the importance of doing well in the high-pressure, high-stakes environment of test day. Your results on this test could have a significant impact on your future, and this guide provides the information and practical advice to help you achieve your full potential on test day.

Your success is our success

We would love to hear from you! If you would like to share the story of your exam success or if you have any questions or comments in regard to our products, please contact us at **800-673-8175** or **support@mometrix.com**.

Thanks again for your business and we wish you continued success!

Sincerely,
The Mometrix Test Preparation Team

Need more help? Check out our flashcards at:
http://mometrixflashcards.com/CDN

Table of Contents

Introduction 1
Secret Key #1 – Plan Big, Study Small 2
Secret Key #2 – Make Your Studying Count 3
Secret Key #3 – Practice the Right Way 4
Secret Key #4 – Pace Yourself 6
Secret Key #5 – Have a Plan for Guessing 7
Test-Taking Strategies 10
Concepts of Kidney Disease 15
    Pathophysiology 15
    Measuring Kidney Function 28
    Complications 30
    Interventions 31
Hemodialysis 46
    Hemodialysis 50
    Complications 64
    Interventions 73
    Education 85
    Medication Administration 87
    Psychological and Sociocultural Interventions 91
    Infection Control 92
    Patient Rights and Regulatory Guidelines 98
Peritoneal Dialysis 100
    Peritoneal Dialysis Complications 104
    Interventions 107
Transplant and Acute Therapies 110
CDN Practice Test 118
Answer Key and Explanations 146
How to Overcome Test Anxiety 171
    Causes of Test Anxiety 171
    Elements of Test Anxiety 172
    Effects of Test Anxiety 172
    Physical Steps for Beating Test Anxiety 173
    Mental Steps for Beating Test Anxiety 174
    Study Strategy 175
    Test Tips 177
    Important Qualification 178
Tell Us Your Story 179

ADDITIONAL BONUS MATERIAL _____ 180

Introduction

Thank you for purchasing this resource! You have made the choice to prepare yourself for a test that could have a huge impact on your future, and this guide is designed to help you be fully ready for test day. Obviously, it's important to have a solid understanding of the test material, but you also need to be prepared for the unique environment and stressors of the test, so that you can perform to the best of your abilities.

For this purpose, the first section that appears in this guide is the **Secret Keys**. We've devoted countless hours to meticulously researching what works and what doesn't, and we've boiled down our findings to the five most impactful steps you can take to improve your performance on the test. We start at the beginning with study planning and move through the preparation process, all the way to the testing strategies that will help you get the most out of what you know when you're finally sitting in front of the test.

We recommend that you start preparing for your test as far in advance as possible. However, if you've bought this guide as a last-minute study resource and only have a few days before your test, we recommend that you skip over the first two Secret Keys since they address a long-term study plan.

If you struggle with **test anxiety**, we strongly encourage you to check out our recommendations for how you can overcome it. Test anxiety is a formidable foe, but it can be beaten, and we want to make sure you have the tools you need to defeat it.

Secret Key #1 – Plan Big, Study Small

There's a lot riding on your performance. If you want to ace this test, you're going to need to keep your skills sharp and the material fresh in your mind. You need a plan that lets you review everything you need to know while still fitting in your schedule. We'll break this strategy down into three categories.

Information Organization

Start with the information you already have: the official test outline. From this, you can make a complete list of all the concepts you need to cover before the test. Organize these concepts into groups that can be studied together, and create a list of any related vocabulary you need to learn so you can brush up on any difficult terms. You'll want to keep this vocabulary list handy once you actually start studying since you may need to add to it along the way.

Time Management

Once you have your set of study concepts, decide how to spread them out over the time you have left before the test. Break your study plan into small, clear goals so you have a manageable task for each day and know exactly what you're doing. Then just focus on one small step at a time. When you manage your time this way, you don't need to spend hours at a time studying. Studying a small block of content for a short period each day helps you retain information better and avoid stressing over how much you have left to do. You can relax knowing that you have a plan to cover everything in time. In order for this strategy to be effective though, you have to start studying early and stick to your schedule. Avoid the exhaustion and futility that comes from last-minute cramming!

Study Environment

The environment you study in has a big impact on your learning. Studying in a coffee shop, while probably more enjoyable, is not likely to be as fruitful as studying in a quiet room. It's important to keep distractions to a minimum. You're only planning to study for a short block of time, so make the most of it. Don't pause to check your phone or get up to find a snack. It's also important to **avoid multitasking**. Research has consistently shown that multitasking will make your studying dramatically less effective. Your study area should also be comfortable and well-lit so you don't have the distraction of straining your eyes or sitting on an uncomfortable chair.

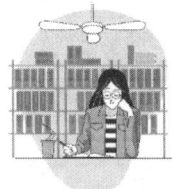

The time of day you study is also important. You want to be rested and alert. Don't wait until just before bedtime. Study when you'll be most likely to comprehend and remember. Even better, if you know what time of day your test will be, set that time aside for study. That way your brain will be used to working on that subject at that specific time and you'll have a better chance of recalling information.

Finally, it can be helpful to team up with others who are studying for the same test. Your actual studying should be done in as isolated an environment as possible, but the work of organizing the information and setting up the study plan can be divided up. In between study sessions, you can discuss with your teammates the concepts that you're all studying and quiz each other on the details. Just be sure that your teammates are as serious about the test as you are. If you find that your study time is being replaced with social time, you might need to find a new team.

Secret Key #2 – Make Your Studying Count

You're devoting a lot of time and effort to preparing for this test, so you want to be absolutely certain it will pay off. This means doing more than just reading the content and hoping you can remember it on test day. It's important to make every minute of study count. There are two main areas you can focus on to make your studying count.

Retention

It doesn't matter how much time you study if you can't remember the material. You need to make sure you are retaining the concepts. To check your retention of the information you're learning, try recalling it at later times with minimal prompting. Try carrying around flashcards and glance at one or two from time to time or ask a friend who's also studying for the test to quiz you.

To enhance your retention, look for ways to put the information into practice so that you can apply it rather than simply recalling it. If you're using the information in practical ways, it will be much easier to remember. Similarly, it helps to solidify a concept in your mind if you're not only reading it to yourself but also explaining it to someone else. Ask a friend to let you teach them about a concept you're a little shaky on (or speak aloud to an imaginary audience if necessary). As you try to summarize, define, give examples, and answer your friend's questions, you'll understand the concepts better and they will stay with you longer. Finally, step back for a big picture view and ask yourself how each piece of information fits with the whole subject. When you link the different concepts together and see them working together as a whole, it's easier to remember the individual components.

Finally, practice showing your work on any multi-step problems, even if you're just studying. Writing out each step you take to solve a problem will help solidify the process in your mind, and you'll be more likely to remember it during the test.

Modality

Modality simply refers to the means or method by which you study. Choosing a study modality that fits your own individual learning style is crucial. No two people learn best in exactly the same way, so it's important to know your strengths and use them to your advantage.

For example, if you learn best by visualization, focus on visualizing a concept in your mind and draw an image or a diagram. Try color-coding your notes, illustrating them, or creating symbols that will trigger your mind to recall a learned concept. If you learn best by hearing or discussing information, find a study partner who learns the same way or read aloud to yourself. Think about how to put the information in your own words. Imagine that you are giving a lecture on the topic and record yourself so you can listen to it later.

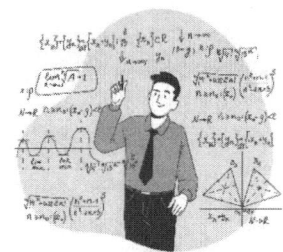

For any learning style, flashcards can be helpful. Organize the information so you can take advantage of spare moments to review. Underline key words or phrases. Use different colors for different categories. Mnemonic devices (such as creating a short list in which every item starts with the same letter) can also help with retention. Find what works best for you and use it to store the information in your mind most effectively and easily.

Secret Key #3 – Practice the Right Way

Your success on test day depends not only on how many hours you put into preparing, but also on whether you prepared the right way. It's good to check along the way to see if your studying is paying off. One of the most effective ways to do this is by taking practice tests to evaluate your progress. Practice tests are useful because they show exactly where you need to improve. Every time you take a practice test, pay special attention to these three groups of questions:

- The questions you got wrong
- The questions you had to guess on, even if you guessed right
- The questions you found difficult or slow to work through

This will show you exactly what your weak areas are, and where you need to devote more study time. Ask yourself why each of these questions gave you trouble. Was it because you didn't understand the material? Was it because you didn't remember the vocabulary? Do you need more repetitions on this type of question to build speed and confidence? Dig into those questions and figure out how you can strengthen your weak areas as you go back to review the material.

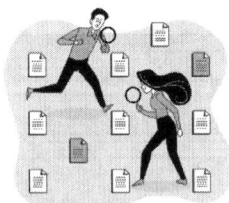

Additionally, many practice tests have a section explaining the answer choices. It can be tempting to read the explanation and think that you now have a good understanding of the concept. However, an explanation likely only covers part of the question's broader context. Even if the explanation makes perfect sense, **go back and investigate** every concept related to the question until you're positive you have a thorough understanding.

As you go along, keep in mind that the practice test is just that: practice. Memorizing these questions and answers will not be very helpful on the actual test because it is unlikely to have any of the same exact questions. If you only know the right answers to the sample questions, you won't be prepared for the real thing. **Study the concepts** until you understand them fully, and then you'll be able to answer any question that shows up on the test.

It's important to wait on the practice tests until you're ready. If you take a test on your first day of study, you may be overwhelmed by the amount of material covered and how much you need to learn. Work up to it gradually.

On test day, you'll need to be prepared for answering questions, managing your time, and using the test-taking strategies you've learned. It's a lot to balance, like a mental marathon that will have a big impact on your future. Like training for a marathon, you'll need to start slowly and work your way up. When test day arrives, you'll be ready.

Start with the strategies you've read in the first two Secret Keys—plan your course and study in the way that works best for you. If you have time, consider using multiple study resources to get different approaches to the same concepts. It can be helpful to see difficult concepts from more than one angle. Then find a good source for practice tests. Many times, the test website will suggest potential study resources or provide sample tests.

Practice Test Strategy

If you're able to find at least three practice tests, we recommend this strategy:

Untimed and Open-Book Practice

Take the first test with no time constraints and with your notes and study guide handy. Take your time and focus on applying the strategies you've learned.

Timed and Open-Book Practice

Take the second practice test open-book as well, but set a timer and practice pacing yourself to finish in time.

Timed and Closed-Book Practice

Take any other practice tests as if it were test day. Set a timer and put away your study materials. Sit at a table or desk in a quiet room, imagine yourself at the testing center, and answer questions as quickly and accurately as possible.

Keep repeating timed and closed-book tests on a regular basis until you run out of practice tests or it's time for the actual test. Your mind will be ready for the schedule and stress of test day, and you'll be able to focus on recalling the material you've learned.

Secret Key #4 – Pace Yourself

Once you're fully prepared for the material on the test, your biggest challenge on test day will be managing your time. Just knowing that the clock is ticking can make you panic even if you have plenty of time left. Work on pacing yourself so you can build confidence against the time constraints of the exam. Pacing is a difficult skill to master, especially in a high-pressure environment, so **practice is vital**.

Set time expectations for your pace based on how much time is available. For example, if a section has 60 questions and the time limit is 30 minutes, you know you have to average 30 seconds or less per question in order to answer them all. Although 30 seconds is the hard limit, set 25 seconds per question as your goal, so you reserve extra time to spend on harder questions. When you budget extra time for the harder questions, you no longer have any reason to stress when those questions take longer to answer.

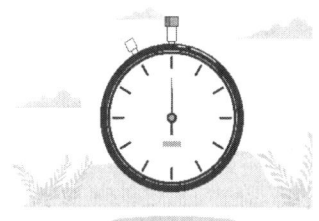

Don't let this time expectation distract you from working through the test at a calm, steady pace, but keep it in mind so you don't spend too much time on any one question. Recognize that taking extra time on one question you don't understand may keep you from answering two that you do understand later in the test. If your time limit for a question is up and you're still not sure of the answer, mark it and move on, and come back to it later if the time and the test format allow. If the testing format doesn't allow you to return to earlier questions, just make an educated guess; then put it out of your mind and move on.

On the easier questions, be careful not to rush. It may seem wise to hurry through them so you have more time for the challenging ones, but it's not worth missing one if you know the concept and just didn't take the time to read the question fully. Work efficiently but make sure you understand the question and have looked at all of the answer choices, since more than one may seem right at first.

Even if you're paying attention to the time, you may find yourself a little behind at some point. You should speed up to get back on track, but do so wisely. Don't panic; just take a few seconds less on each question until you're caught up. Don't guess without thinking, but do look through the answer choices and eliminate any you know are wrong. If you can get down to two choices, it is often worthwhile to guess from those. Once you've chosen an answer, move on and don't dwell on any that you skipped or had to hurry through. If a question was taking too long, chances are it was one of the harder ones, so you weren't as likely to get it right anyway.

On the other hand, if you find yourself getting ahead of schedule, it may be beneficial to slow down a little. The more quickly you work, the more likely you are to make a careless mistake that will affect your score. You've budgeted time for each question, so don't be afraid to spend that time. Practice an efficient but careful pace to get the most out of the time you have.

Secret Key #5 – Have a Plan for Guessing

When you're taking the test, you may find yourself stuck on a question. Some of the answer choices seem better than others, but you don't see the one answer choice that is obviously correct. What do you do?

The scenario described above is very common, yet most test takers have not effectively prepared for it. Developing and practicing a plan for guessing may be one of the single most effective uses of your time as you get ready for the exam.

In developing your plan for guessing, there are three questions to address:

- When should you start the guessing process?
- How should you narrow down the choices?
- Which answer should you choose?

When to Start the Guessing Process

Unless your plan for guessing is to select C every time (which, despite its merits, is not what we recommend), you need to leave yourself enough time to apply your answer elimination strategies. Since you have a limited amount of time for each question, that means that if you're going to give yourself the best shot at guessing correctly, you have to decide quickly whether or not you will guess.

Of course, the best-case scenario is that you don't have to guess at all, so first, see if you can answer the question based on your knowledge of the subject and basic reasoning skills. Focus on the key words in the question and try to jog your memory of related topics. Give yourself a chance to bring the knowledge to mind, but once you realize that you don't have (or you can't access) the knowledge you need to answer the question, it's time to start the guessing process.

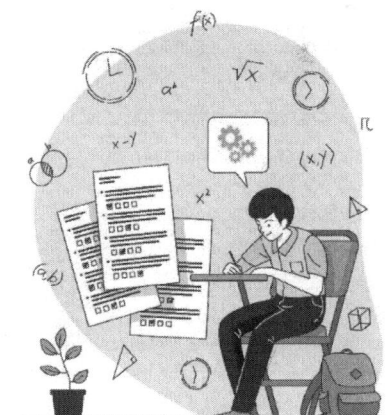

It's almost always better to start the guessing process too early than too late. It only takes a few seconds to remember something and answer the question from knowledge. Carefully eliminating wrong answer choices takes longer. Plus, going through the process of eliminating answer choices can actually help jog your memory.

Summary: Start the guessing process as soon as you decide that you can't answer the question based on your knowledge.

How to Narrow Down the Choices

The next chapter in this book (**Test-Taking Strategies**) includes a wide range of strategies for how to approach questions and how to look for answer choices to eliminate. You will definitely want to read those carefully, practice them, and figure out which ones work best for you. Here though, we're going to address a mindset rather than a particular strategy.

Your odds of guessing an answer correctly depend on how many options you are choosing from.

Number of options left	5	4	3	2	1
Odds of guessing correctly	20%	25%	33%	50%	100%

You can see from this chart just how valuable it is to be able to eliminate incorrect answers and make an educated guess, but there are two things that many test takers do that cause them to miss out on the benefits of guessing:

- Accidentally eliminating the correct answer
- Selecting an answer based on an impression

We'll look at the first one here, and the second one in the next section.

To avoid accidentally eliminating the correct answer, we recommend a thought exercise called **the $5 challenge**. In this challenge, you only eliminate an answer choice from contention if you are willing to bet $5 on it being wrong. Why $5? Five dollars is a small but not insignificant amount of money. It's an amount you could afford to lose but wouldn't want to throw away. And while losing

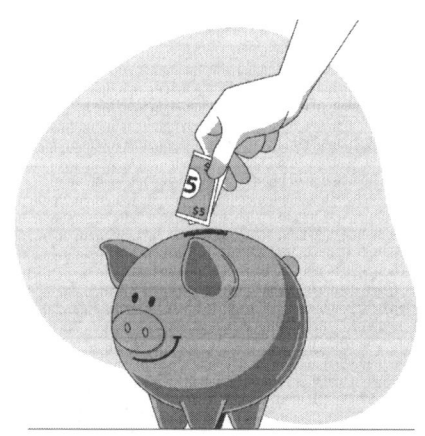

$5 once might not hurt too much, doing it twenty times will set you back $100. In the same way, each small decision you make—eliminating a choice here, guessing on a question there—won't by itself impact your score very much, but when you put them all together, they can make a big difference. By holding each answer choice elimination decision to a higher standard, you can reduce the risk of accidentally eliminating the correct answer.

The $5 challenge can also be applied in a positive sense: If you are willing to bet $5 that an answer choice *is* correct, go ahead and mark it as correct.

Summary: Only eliminate an answer choice if you are willing to bet $5 that it is wrong.

Which Answer to Choose

You're taking the test. You've run into a hard question and decided you'll have to guess. You've eliminated all the answer choices you're willing to bet $5 on. Now you have to pick an answer. Why do we even need to talk about this? Why can't you just pick whichever one you feel like when the time comes?

The answer to these questions is that if you don't come into the test with a plan, you'll rely on your impression to select an answer choice, and if you do that, you risk falling into a trap. The test writers know that everyone who takes their test will be guessing on some of the questions, so they intentionally write wrong answer choices to seem plausible. You still have to pick an answer though, and if the wrong answer choices are designed to look right, how can you ever be sure that you're not falling for their trap? The best solution we've found to this dilemma is to take the decision out of your hands entirely. Here is the process we recommend:

Once you've eliminated any choices that you are confident (willing to bet $5) are wrong, select the first remaining choice as your answer.

Whether you choose to select the first remaining choice, the second, or the last, the important thing is that you use some preselected standard. Using this approach guarantees that you will not be enticed into selecting an answer choice that looks right, because you are not basing your decision on how the answer choices look.

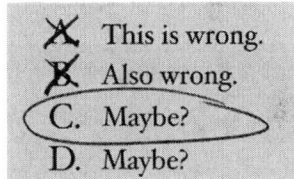

This is not meant to make you question your knowledge. Instead, it is to help you recognize the difference between your knowledge and your impressions. There's a huge difference between thinking an answer is right because of what you know, and thinking an answer is right because it looks or sounds like it should be right.

Summary: To ensure that your selection is appropriately random, make a predetermined selection from among all answer choices you have not eliminated.

Test-Taking Strategies

This section contains a list of test-taking strategies that you may find helpful as you work through the test. By taking what you know and applying logical thought, you can maximize your chances of answering any question correctly!

It is very important to realize that every question is different and every person is different: no single strategy will work on every question, and no single strategy will work for every person. That's why we've included all of them here, so you can try them out and determine which ones work best for different types of questions and which ones work best for you.

Question Strategies

✓ READ CAREFULLY

Read the question and the answer choices carefully. Don't miss the question because you misread the terms. You have plenty of time to read each question thoroughly and make sure you understand what is being asked. Yet a happy medium must be attained, so don't waste too much time. You must read carefully and efficiently.

✓ CONTEXTUAL CLUES

Look for contextual clues. If the question includes a word you are not familiar with, look at the immediate context for some indication of what the word might mean. Contextual clues can often give you all the information you need to decipher the meaning of an unfamiliar word. Even if you can't determine the meaning, you may be able to narrow down the possibilities enough to make a solid guess at the answer to the question.

✓ PREFIXES

If you're having trouble with a word in the question or answer choices, try dissecting it. Take advantage of every clue that the word might include. Prefixes and suffixes can be a huge help. Usually, they allow you to determine a basic meaning. *Pre-* means before, *post-* means after, *pro-* is positive, *de-* is negative. From prefixes and suffixes, you can get an idea of the general meaning of the word and try to put it into context.

✓ HEDGE WORDS

Watch out for critical hedge words, such as *likely, may, can, sometimes, often, almost, mostly, usually, generally, rarely,* and *sometimes.* Question writers insert these hedge phrases to cover every possibility. Often an answer choice will be wrong simply because it leaves no room for exception. Be on guard for answer choices that have definitive words such as *exactly* and *always*.

✓ SWITCHBACK WORDS

Stay alert for *switchbacks*. These are the words and phrases frequently used to alert you to shifts in thought. The most common switchback words are *but, although,* and *however*. Others include *nevertheless, on the other hand, even though, while, in spite of, despite,* and *regardless of*. Switchback words are important to catch because they can change the direction of the question or an answer choice.

ⓘ Face Value

When in doubt, use common sense. Accept the situation in the problem at face value. Don't read too much into it. These problems will not require you to make wild assumptions. If you have to go beyond creativity and warp time or space in order to have an answer choice fit the question, then you should move on and consider the other answer choices. These are normal problems rooted in reality. The applicable relationship or explanation may not be readily apparent, but it is there for you to figure out. Use your common sense to interpret anything that isn't clear.

Answer Choice Strategies

ⓘ Answer Selection

The most thorough way to pick an answer choice is to identify and eliminate wrong answers until only one is left, then confirm it is the correct answer. Sometimes an answer choice may immediately seem right, but be careful. The test writers will usually put more than one reasonable answer choice on each question, so take a second to read all of them and make sure that the other choices are not equally obvious. As long as you have time left, it is better to read every answer choice than to pick the first one that looks right without checking the others.

ⓘ Answer Choice Families

An answer choice family consists of two (in rare cases, three) answer choices that are very similar in construction and cannot all be true at the same time. If you see two answer choices that are direct opposites or parallels, one of them is usually the correct answer. For instance, if one answer choice says that quantity x increases and another either says that quantity x decreases (opposite) or says that quantity y increases (parallel), then those answer choices would fall into the same family. An answer choice that doesn't match the construction of the answer choice family is more likely to be incorrect. Most questions will not have answer choice families, but when they do appear, you should be prepared to recognize them.

ⓘ Eliminate Answers

Eliminate answer choices as soon as you realize they are wrong, but make sure you consider all possibilities. If you are eliminating answer choices and realize that the last one you are left with is also wrong, don't panic. Start over and consider each choice again. There may be something you missed the first time that you will realize on the second pass.

ⓘ Avoid Fact Traps

Don't be distracted by an answer choice that is factually true but doesn't answer the question. You are looking for the choice that answers the question. Stay focused on what the question is asking for so you don't accidentally pick an answer that is true but incorrect. Always go back to the question and make sure the answer choice you've selected actually answers the question and is not merely a true statement.

ⓘ Extreme Statements

In general, you should avoid answers that put forth extreme actions as standard practice or proclaim controversial ideas as established fact. An answer choice that states the "process should be used in certain situations, if…" is much more likely to be correct than one that states the "process should be discontinued completely." The first is a calm rational statement and doesn't even make a definitive, uncompromising stance, using a hedge word *if* to provide wiggle room, whereas the second choice is far more extreme.

⌀ Benchmark

As you read through the answer choices and you come across one that seems to answer the question well, mentally select that answer choice. This is not your final answer, but it's the one that will help you evaluate the other answer choices. The one that you selected is your benchmark or standard for judging each of the other answer choices. Every other answer choice must be compared to your benchmark. That choice is correct until proven otherwise by another answer choice beating it. If you find a better answer, then that one becomes your new benchmark. Once you've decided that no other choice answers the question as well as your benchmark, you have your final answer.

⌀ Predict the Answer

Before you even start looking at the answer choices, it is often best to try to predict the answer. When you come up with the answer on your own, it is easier to avoid distractions and traps because you will know exactly what to look for. The right answer choice is unlikely to be word-for-word what you came up with, but it should be a close match. Even if you are confident that you have the right answer, you should still take the time to read each option before moving on.

General Strategies

⌀ Tough Questions

If you are stumped on a problem or it appears too hard or too difficult, don't waste time. Move on! Remember though, if you can quickly check for obviously incorrect answer choices, your chances of guessing correctly are greatly improved. Before you completely give up, at least try to knock out a couple of possible answers. Eliminate what you can and then guess at the remaining answer choices before moving on.

⌀ Check Your Work

Since you will probably not know every term listed and the answer to every question, it is important that you get credit for the ones that you do know. Don't miss any questions through careless mistakes. If at all possible, try to take a second to look back over your answer selection and make sure you've selected the correct answer choice and haven't made a costly careless mistake (such as marking an answer choice that you didn't mean to mark). This quick double check should more than pay for itself in caught mistakes for the time it costs.

⌀ Pace Yourself

It's easy to be overwhelmed when you're looking at a page full of questions; your mind is confused and full of random thoughts, and the clock is ticking down faster than you would like. Calm down and maintain the pace that you have set for yourself. Especially as you get down to the last few minutes of the test, don't let the small numbers on the clock make you panic. As long as you are on track by monitoring your pace, you are guaranteed to have time for each question.

⌀ Don't Rush

It is very easy to make errors when you are in a hurry. Maintaining a fast pace in answering questions is pointless if it makes you miss questions that you would have gotten right otherwise. Test writers like to include distracting information and wrong answers that seem right. Taking a little extra time to avoid careless mistakes can make all the difference in your test score. Find a pace that allows you to be confident in the answers that you select.

⊘ Keep Moving

Panicking will not help you pass the test, so do your best to stay calm and keep moving. Taking deep breaths and going through the answer elimination steps you practiced can help to break through a stress barrier and keep your pace.

Final Notes

The combination of a solid foundation of content knowledge and the confidence that comes from practicing your plan for applying that knowledge is the key to maximizing your performance on test day. As your foundation of content knowledge is built up and strengthened, you'll find that the strategies included in this chapter become more and more effective in helping you quickly sift through the distractions and traps of the test to isolate the correct answer.

Now that you're preparing to move forward into the test content chapters of this book, be sure to keep your goal in mind. As you read, think about how you will be able to apply this information on the test. If you've already seen sample questions for the test and you have an idea of the question format and style, try to come up with questions of your own that you can answer based on what you're reading. This will give you valuable practice applying your knowledge in the same ways you can expect to on test day.

Good luck and good studying!

Concepts of Kidney Disease

Pathophysiology

FUNCTIONS OF NORMAL KIDNEYS
Normal kidneys perform several functions including the following:

- Excretion of waste products of metabolism, including urea, uric acid, and water
- Maintenance of acid/base balance (pH)
- Regulation of plasma volume and blood pressure
- Maintenance of electrolyte balance
- Production (synthesis) of hormones, including erythropoietin (which stimulates erythrocyte production in response to low levels of O_2), renin (which regulates aldosterone), and calcitriol (which promotes the absorption of calcium)
- Reception of hormones, including antidiuretic hormone (ADH) produced by the pituitary, which enhances water reabsorption; aldosterone (from the adrenal cortex), which causes the kidneys to retain water and sodium (increasing the b/p); and parathyroid hormone (produced by the parathyroid glands), which increases the calcium: phosphate ratio and results in an increase in calcium in the blood.

CIRCULATION OF KIDNEYS
The kidneys receive up to 25% of resting cardiac output. These highly vascular organs process an average of 1000 ml/min of blood. Circulation to each kidney begins with the renal artery, which branches from the abdominal aorta. The renal artery divides into interlobar arteries, which in turn supply the arcuate arteries. Interlobular arteries branch from the arcuates and further divide into afferent arterioles, which then become glomerular capillaries. The glomerular capillaries then merge to form efferent arterioles that disperse into vasa recta and peritubular capillaries.

- The vasa recta (straight arterioles) and their branches surround the loops of Henle of the juxtamedullary nephrons in the renal medulla, where they function to maintain the concentration gradient of the urine.
- The tiny peritubular capillaries lie adjacent to the nephrons permitting tubular secretion and reabsorption to take place.

CHRONIC KIDNEY DISEASE
According to the National Kidney Foundation, chronic kidney disease is defined as those patients with glomerular filtration rates of less than 60 ml/min/1.73 m² for greater than 3 months. The reasoning behind this is that at a GFR of less than 60, approximately half of the nephrons have been damaged. This is also the GFR where manifestations of chronic kidney disease begin to manifest including anemia, early bone disease, and establishes an increased risk for coronary artery disease.

STAGES
The five stages of chronic kidney disease are listed and defined below:

- Stage I—Glomerular filtration rate > 90 ml/min/1.73 m²
- Stage II—Glomerular filtration rate between 60 – 90 ml/min/1.73 m²
- Stage III—Glomerular filtration rate between 30 – 60 ml/min/1.73 m²

- Stage IV—Glomerular filtration rate between 15 – 30 ml/min/1.73 m²
- Stage V—Glomerular filtration rate <15 ml/min/1.73 m² (needs dialysis)

SCREENING

Screening for CKD is necessary for any patient considered in the high-risk category. Kidney function and an evaluation of proteinuria are both important in assessing a patient for CKD. Since diabetics are at high risk for developing CKD, the American Diabetes Association (ADA) recommends that all patients diagnosed with type 2 diabetes be tested for microalbuminuria at the time of diagnosis. Type 1 diabetics should be tested 5 years after the initial evaluation. Any patient with hypertension or heart disease or who is in any other high-risk group should have routine examinations for kidney involvement. The dipstick test for albumin and blood cells is the first step in analyzing the patient for kidney disease. If positive for albumin, the next step is a protein-creatinine ratio test. If the dipstick is positive for blood or white cells, a more comprehensive microscopic analysis needs to be done.

RISK FACTORS

The major risk factors for chronic kidney disease include:

- diabetes mellitus
- hypertension
- hyperlipidemia
- smoking

These are preventable and very treatable causes of both initiating and progressing kidney disease. They are also the most widely prevalent and present the greatest risk to public health. Other less common risk factors include:

- autoimmune diseases (chiefly systemic lupus erythematosus)
- chronic urinary tract infections
- age, renal stones
- systemic infections
- family history

POLYCYSTIC KIDNEY DISEASE AS A CAUSE

Polycystic kidney disease is the most common genetic condition that can cause renal disease. It is usually inherited in an autosomal dominant fashion, though there are some recessive patterns of inheritance. The usual disease course is one where renal failure develops in young persons between 25-35 years of age. The only treatment is renal replacement therapy and most patients require transplants. It is characterized by large kidney sizes with huge cysts that can often be palpated on physical exam. There are no known treatments that can effectively slow the progression of the disease.

METABOLIC ACIDOSIS

The kidneys are involved in excreting broken down proteins. Proteins break down into their component parts, which are amino acids. Amino acids are, in fact, acids. They are largely buffered in the bloodstream via the presence of the ubiquitous base bicarbonate. When renal failure ensues, the ability to excrete amino acids is hindered. With amino acid build up, the bicarbonate buffer is also exhausted. Therefore, the amino acid build up contributes to the acidosis present in all patients with chronic kidney disease. Renal replacement therapy with appropriate dialysate solutions aids in eliminating the acidosis. Thus, before each dialysis treatment patients are acidotic. Following dialysis, patients should ideally return to neutrality or a pH of 7.4.

Effects on Neurological System

Most patients suffer neurological consequences from chronic uremia. The uremic syndrome can cause dementia marked by incoherent speech, seizures and EEG changes. The precise etiology of uremia-induced dementia has yet to be elucidated. Another less common cause of dementia is chronic aluminum exposure. Aluminum has been shown to accumulate in patients with chronic kidney disease. The most common source of aluminum used to be phosphate binders. Although aluminum induced dementia is rare today, it is still seen with aluminum coming from contaminated water supplies. Another neurologic consequence of dialysis is neuropathy. The exact mechanism is unknown but the neuropathy presents as numbness or burning of the extremities, reduced vibratory sense and twitching. Inadequate dialysis has been implicated as a possible cause for the neuropathy but more research is needed.

Effects on Joints

Patients on renal replacement therapy frequently have elevated uric acid levels. Uric acid is implicated in causing gout. Gout is a disease where uric acid crystals precipitate and deposit into joints. The most common joints involved include the distal joint of the great toe, elbows and knees. Another disease of the joints that is frequently seen in dialysis patients is pseudogout. Pseudogout is arthritis where calcium pyrophosphate crystals deposit into joints. Patients will complain of pain and inflammation at the wrist, fingers, back of the hands and knees. Finally, β2 microglobulin amyloidosis causes joint pains and hemarthrosis (blood in joints). It affects nearly any joint in the body.

Effects on Reproductive Endocrine System

Women on dialysis rarely menstruate if at all. The ability to ovulate has also come into question. Uremia seems to interfere with the normal hormonal balance and appears to quell ovulation. In men, uremia has been shown to decrease sperm production. Furthermore, libido in both sexes is markedly reduced. The exact etiology for the described endocrine phenomena is unknown. They seem to be another piece of the puzzle in the constellation of symptoms, which contribute to the uremic syndrome.

Effects on Respiratory System

Patients with chronic kidney disease do not adequately excrete water. Thus, patients on dialysis are frequently volume overloaded. When the excess water is combined with weakened cardiac muscle, pulmonary edema occurs. Patients on dialysis frequently battle pulmonary edema and the best therapy is dialysis with increased filtration or transmembrane pressures. The elevated transmembrane pressure will forcibly push the excess water through the dialyzer under convective forces.

Effects on Cardiovascular System

Chronic kidney disease is frequently associated with hypertension and fluid retention. Hypertension and fluid retention is taxing to the heart and can lead to myocardial wall thickening called left ventricular hypertrophy. Left ventricular hypertrophy is an increase in the size of the left ventricle secondary to increased stress placed on the heart from hypertension and excess fluid. Chronic left ventricular hypertrophy can lead to heart failure. Ace inhibitors are the drug of choice in treating patients with left ventricular hypertrophy and those who have progressed to congestive heart failure. Other effects of renal failure on the cardiovascular system include coronary artery calcification and pericarditis. The heart is surrounded by a sac, which can become inflamed and fluid filled. When that happens, it is known as pericarditis. Pericarditis frequently presents as chest pain with a friction rub heard on auscultation. It is an indication for urgent dialysis.

Effects on Gastrointestinal System

Patients with chronic kidney disease frequently complain of decreased appetite and metallic tastes in their mouths. Both are due to complications of uremia with little treatment options. Another common gastrointestinal issue is one of internal bleeding. The mucosa of the gastrointestinal tract is more friable because of the systems inability to coagulate (platelet dysfunction). Thus, patients on dialysis will frequently have gastrointestinal bleeding. Proton pump inhibitors are one measure to help aid in the healing of any gastric or peptic ulcers noted. Lower gastrointestinal bleeds may require colonoscopy or bowel resection depending on the extent of the bleeding.

EFFECTS ON INTEGUMENTARY SYSTEM

Foremost, ecchymosis is frequently seen on the skin of most patients. This is due to a combination of frequent blood draws and platelet dysfunction. Also seen is skin pallor, which is secondary to anemia of chronic disease. Finally, patients with uremic syndrome symptoms may experience pruritus for reasons unknown. They will frequently itch and scars and erythema are frequently noted.

ESRD

EFFECTS ON IMMUNE SYSTEM

In the early stages of the immune deficiency, uremic toxins are thought to play an important role while the dialysis procedure itself leads to a state of chronic inflammation. Infection is the second most common cause of death in ESRD patients with cardiovascular mortality ranking number one. Immunodepression contributes to the high incidence of infection in this group. The combination of reduced WBC count and poor granulocytic response to infection results in decreased bacteriocidal capability. Other contributing factors are malnutrition, frequency of cannulation, and invasive procedures. The elevated uremic level has an effect on the body's ability to develop a fever as a response to infection. The ESRD patient may present with a subnormal body temperature, so care must be taken to assess the patient's response to infection.

EFFECTS ON ENDOCRINE SYSTEM

Endocrine system effects in the ESRD patients include the following:

- Insulin production
- Parathyroid hormone levels disorder
- Increased plasma norepinephrine
- Inconsistent epinephrine levels
- Increased aldosterone
- Elevated levels of glucagon (pancreatic hormone used for carbohydrate metabolism) and gastrin (stimulates the secretion of gastric acid), which occurs as a consequence of renal metabolism clearance
- Hypothyroidism
- Low response to thyroid-releasing hormone (TRH) with mostly normal response to thyroid-stimulating hormone (TSH)
- Increased growth hormone and prolactin
- Abnormal production of estrogen, progesterone, or testosterone
- Elevated luteinizing hormone (LH) in both sexes

EFFECTS ON HEMATOLOGIC SYSTEM

The most common problem is anemia. Kidney failure leads to a decrease in erythropoietin production, which leads to less red blood cell production by the bone marrow. Anemia is treated with supplemental erythropoietin and iron. Another frequently encountered hematologic abnormality is platelet dysfunction. Platelets are important in clotting and help prevent excess blood loss. Yet, uremia alters platelet function and bleeding diathesis is problematic. Hemodialysis patients require frequent blood draws, which leaves them with bruising and hematomas. Moreover, gastrointestinal bleeding is concerning for the body is incapable of adequately quelling the loss of blood. Proton pump inhibitors aid in alleviating blood loss secondary to gastric ulcers.

CAUSES OF CHRONIC KIDNEY DISEASE IN CHILDREN

The most common causes of chronic kidney disease in children are congenital anomalies. These include:

- Obstructive uropathy
- Reflux nephropathy
- Renal dysplasia
- Autosomal recessive polycystic kidney disease
- Other hereditary diseases

Acquired forms of chronic kidney disease include glomerular diseases such as focal segmental glomerulosclerosis and membranoproliferative glomerulonephritis.

PRERENAL FAILURE

PATHOPHYSIOLOGY

Prerenal failure is due to an inadequate blood pressure reaching the renal arteries. The renal arteries respond to low blood pressure by releasing the local hormone renin. Renin causes the release of angiotensin I which travels to the lungs and causes the release of the potent angiotensin II. Angiotensin II causes vasoconstriction of the renal arteries, which will help elevate the pressure delivered to the kidneys. It is important to know that ace inhibitors act to block the converting enzyme, which produces angiotensin II. While this may seem counterintuitive, it is important to differentiate the physiology of acute renal failure and normal renal function. Under normal physiologic conditions, ace inhibitors are helpful in preventing the progression of renal failure. However, during acute renal failure, ace inhibitors are contraindicated.

MAJOR CAUSES

Prerenal failure results from anything that causes decreased blood flow to the kidneys. This includes:

- Dehydration
- Congestive heart failure
- Liver cirrhosis
- Septic shock
- Cardiogenic shock
- Anaphylactic shock
- Medications

Dehydration results from excess intravascular water loss secondary to exercise, diarrhea, and vomiting. Congestive heart failure and liver cirrhosis deliver less blood volume to the kidneys. The former is due to an ineffective pump (the heart) and the latter is due to third spacing (fluids leaving the vascular system and entering the interstitium). Septic shock is found with blood born pathogens particularly gram-negative bacteria. Cardiogenic shock results when the heart is incapable of pumping blood effectively usually from an acute infarction. Anaphylactic shock is secondary to the release of histamines in response to an allergen. Medications causing prerenal failure include diuretics and ace inhibitors.

<u>CONGESTIVE HEART FAILURE AND DEHYDRATION:</u> Congestive heart failure occurs when cardiac muscle fails to pump blood effectively. This can be due to either an inability of cardiac muscle to contract (systolic dysfunction) or relax (diastolic dysfunction). Both mechanisms lead to ineffective circulating blood volumes reaching the kidney.

Dehydration by any mechanism results in a loss of effective circulating volume. The major reasons for dehydration include:

- Exercise
- Diarrhea
- Vomiting
- Medications, chiefly diuretics

The effect of both instances is acute renal failure secondary to prerenal azotemia. The kidney responds by releasing renin, a local hormone which causes the release of angiotensin I. Angiotensin I travels to the lungs and is converted to angiotensin II which is a potent vasoconstrictor. Angiotensin II will cause the renal arteries to constrict and increase the blood pressure at the level of the kidneys.

LIVER CIRRHOSIS AND SEPTIC SHOCK: Liver cirrhosis is a very common cause of acute renal failure in patients with chronic liver disease. The mechanism is as follows: fluid accumulates in the interstitium and lower extremities due to the lack of serum albumin. The liver produces albumin. Albumin is the chief protein responsible for providing the oncotic pressure needed to retain fluid in the vascular system. Without albumin, fluid will traverse the blood vessels and enter the interstitium via osmosis.

Septic shock is caused by an overwhelming infection in the bloodstream, most commonly from gram negative bacteria. The immune system is overwhelmed by the infectious agent and the response is a loss of vasomotor tone. The arteries vasodilate to the point of causing hypotension. The decrease in blood pressure leads to an ineffective volume reaching the kidneys.

The effect of both conditions is acute renal failure secondary to prerenal azotemia.

CARDIOGENIC SHOCK AND ANAPHYLACTIC SHOCK: Cardiogenic shock is not unlike congestive heart failure in its mechanism for causing acute renal failure. Cardiogenic shock is due to a myocardium which does not pump effectively. However, unlike with congestive heart failure, cardiogenic shock is usually an acute event. The most common cause of cardiogenic shock is a large myocardial infarction. When the heart does not pump effectively, the systemic blood pressure falls and the kidneys sense this drop in pressure.

Anaphylactic shock is due to the body's response to an allergen. Unlike allergies causing nasal congestion or hives, this response is far more severe. The release of histamine from the body causes the blood vessels to vasodilate and results in hypotension. The hypotension causes a decrease in blood pressure at the level of the kidney. The effect of both conditions is acute renal failure secondary to prerenal azotemia.

ACE INHIBITORS: Ace inhibitors are commonly used to prevent the progression of renal disease in patients with chronic kidney disease. Their mechanism of action is such that they can also precipitate acute renal failure. When the kidney senses a decrease in blood pressure, it responds by releasing renin, a local hormone which causes the release of angiotensin I. Angiotensin I travels to the lungs and is converted to angiotensin II which is a potent vasoconstrictor. Angiotensin II will cause the renal arteries to constrict and increase the blood pressure at the level of the kidneys. Ace-inhibitors act by blocking the enzyme angiotensin converting enzyme. This enzyme is the key step in the conversion of angiotensin to angiotensin II. While ace-inhibitors have been effective in stopping proteinuria and progression of chronic kidney disease, they can also precipitate acute renal failure by the aforementioned mechanism.

INTRINSIC RENAL FAILURE

Intrinsic renal failure is secondary to directly injury to the renal parenchyma. Specifically, the damage can occur to the renal tubules, interstitium, glomeruli and renal arteries and veins. Damage that occurs to the interstitium includes those caused by medications, chiefly non-steroidal anti-inflammatory drugs and antibiotics (penicillins and aminoglycosides). The list of medications causing renal damage is too exhaustive to list but the most common include lithium, chemotherapies, heavy metals and amphotericin (antifungal). Glomerular damage is secondary to systemic lupus erythematosus, glomerulonephritis and various forms of vasculitis. Renal arteries and veins are damaged by embolic phenomena from atrial fibrillation and endocarditis. Other causes of intrinsic renal failure include ischemia and damage from radiocontrast administered during angiograms and cat scans.

INFECTIONS THAT CAN SCAR KIDNEYS

An infection of the kidney and renal pelvis is termed pyelonephritis. This occurs when bacteria, usually from the bowel, ascend through the lower urinary tract. Once in the kidney, the infection may lead to fibrosis and scarring. Fluoroquinolones (ciprofloxacin), amoxicillin, cephalosporin, and trimethoprim are the drugs of choice for treatment of these infections. If leukocytosis and a high fever are present, IV administration of the antibiotic may be indicated. *Mycobacterium tuberculosis* cause renal tuberculosis as a secondary site to the primary lung infection. Caseation, in which dead tissue decays and forms a dry mass, occurs in the tubercular lesions. The kidneys are scarred, calcified, and permanently damaged. Findings may include dysuria, hematuria, sterile pyuria, albuminuria, and urgency. The client may complain of suprapubic pain, increased urination, and fever. Diagnosis is by culture of acid-fast bacillus, cystoscopy, needle biopsy, or imaging. Renal tuberculosis often remains dormant for several years after the patient's pulmonary infection before causing any symptoms.

POST RENAL FAILURE

Post renal failure results when there is an obstruction of urinary flow out of the kidneys. The most common causes include prostatic hypertrophy, crystal disease and extrarenal causes of ureteral obstruction. When the prostate enlarges, it can block urinary flow as it passes through the urethra. Crystal disease includes kidney stones secondary to uric acid, calcium or struvite stones. The crystals deposit in the distal tubules of the kidney and cause tubular damage resulting in an inability to generate adequate urine flow. Extrarenal causes of ureteral obstruction include retroperitoneal fibrosis, bladder cancer and colon cancer (the tumor enlarges from the colon and compresses the urethra).

INFECTIOUS CAUSES OF RENAL FAILURE

The most common infectious cause of renal failure is bacterial. Pyelonephritis is inflammation of the kidneys secondary to an infectious agent, usually bacterial. Treatment includes use of broad-spectrum antibiotics, usually quinolones. Other less common causes include mycobacterium tuberculosis and fungal infections. Both have been known to cause renal failure in immunocompromised patients and those with HIV. Finally, a rare but interesting cause of renal failure is post streptococcal glomerulonephritis. Patients will have strep throat and two weeks later present with renal failure and hematuria. The renal failure is caused by streptococcal antigens forming immune complexes that deposit in the glomerulus. This immune complex causes the glomerulonephritis and renal failure ensues. The renal failure is usually self-limited and patients recover full kidney function after approximately a two-week course.

PKD

Polycystic kidney disease (PKD) is the third leading cause of renal failure. It is a genetic disease, and both sexes are equally likely to be affected. Dominant genes cause most cases of PKD with one rare type originating from a recessive gene. In the recessive gene type of PKD, the disease becomes symptomatic early in childhood and usually has a poor prognosis. In the more common form, the autosomal dominant, symptoms may present in early (50% develop cysts before age 18) to mid-adulthood. Fluid-filled cysts replace normal kidney tissue, as these cysts grow; they crowd the healthy tissue until kidney function deteriorates.

Symptoms may include the following:

1. Flank or low-back pain
2. Urinary tract infections
3. Hematuria
4. Severe hypertension
5. Fatigue
6. Nausea
7. Kidney stones with accompanying pain
8. Increase in abdominal girth Infection of the kidneys may further weaken the kidneys ability to function. Nephrectomy may be the only option for the painful, chronically infected kidney.

In addition to cysts in the kidneys, PKD may cause cysts to form in the liver, pancreas, testes, ovaries and spleen. Brain aneurysms have been found in approximately 10% of PKD cases.

NEPHROTIC SYNDROME

Nephrotic syndrome is a myriad of clinical findings that result in massive losses of protein through the kidney due to damaged, leaky glomeruli. When the protein level in the blood declines, fluid shifts into the tissues resulting in edema. Patients with nephrotic syndrome are at an increased risk for thrombosis and infection. Pitting edema in the legs, puffiness in the periorbital area upon awakening, abdominal ascites, and pulmonary edema may be seen with this syndrome. The high protein level may cause the urine to appear 'foamy'. Dietary recommendations include a low sodium diet, avoidance of saturated fats, monitoring of fluid intake, and increased fruits and vegetables. Treatment depends upon the underlying cause of the condition. Immunosuppressants, diabetic blood glucose control, and hypertension medications to maintain blood pressure levels are used to treat the underlying disease processes that lead to the nephrotic syndrome.

Nephrotic syndrome is defined by the following: heavy proteinuria (>3.5 gms over 24 hours), hyperlipidemia, hypercoagulability, edema with frequent hypertension. The edema is caused by the excessive protein loss in the urine. The lack of protein in the serum causes fluids to shift into the interstitial and intracellular spaces. Thus, patients with nephrotic syndrome retain a lot of fluid in dependent areas. It is caused by a myriad of conditions including diabetes, glomerulonephritis, lupus and hypertension. Treatment is targeted at treating the underlying condition with use of diuretics and ace inhibitors. The former is to relieve excess water retention and the latter is to slow the progression of protein loss and further kidney damage.

AMYLOIDOSIS

Amyloidosis is a rare disorder and is either primary or secondary. Primary amyloidosis is caused by deposition of light chains from antibodies. These proteins cause organ dysfunction and lead to renal failure. Primary amyloidosis carries a poor prognosis and treatments are not curative. Secondary amyloidosis is a more chronic and progressive condition where proteins deposit in most any organ system. Again, these proteins cause organ dysfunction and they can deposit in the heart, liver, skin and kidneys. Treatment options are also limited and renal failure is treated with replacement therapy. The only known agents to slow the progression of renal failure from amyloidosis are ace inhibitors.

RENAL CELL CARCINOMA

Renal cell carcinoma is cancer of the kidney as the name implies. It is usually diagnosed in patients over 50 who present with painless hematuria. Renal cell cancers also secrete erythropoietin. Thus, checking erythropoietin levels is a diagnostic clue. CAT scans and ultrasounds are used to locate the tumor and biopsies are performed to grade the cancer. Treatment consists of a nephrectomy with attempts to preserve the other kidney. However, if both kidneys are affected (rare), then bilateral nephrectomies are indicated. Renal replacement therapy is offered to those who require it.

RENAL ARTERY STENOSIS

Renal artery stenosis is a condition where there is a significant narrowing of the renal arteries. There are two primary causes:

- Fibromuscular dysplasia (more common in young women)
- Atherosclerosis

Fibromuscular dysplasia is caused by smooth muscle build up in the renal arteries causing a narrowing of the lumen. Atherosclerosis is the same mechanism of luminal narrowing as found in patients with coronary artery disease. Patients with renal artery stenosis present with severe hypertension and often develop renal failure (from a lack of adequate blood supply). Treatment includes stents and renal artery bypass surgery. Ace inhibitors are a relative contraindication in patients with renal artery stenosis.

ALBUMIN

In ESRD patients, serum albumin levels are important in predicting morbidity and mortality. Albumin is the most prevalent protein found in plasma. It has the role of transporting the smaller molecules of drugs, calcium and bilirubin in the bloodstream. It helps maintain the fluid volume in the blood vessels. This form of protein is an accurate gauge for the nutritional status of the ESRD patient. The levels are a direct reflection of the diet protein intake, which may be insufficient due to the patient's lack of appetite. The desired range for serum albumin in the ESRD patient is greater than 4.0g/dL. Symptoms of low serum albumin (hypoalbuminemia) include edema, weight loss, muscle wasting, fatigue, and hypotension. The risks for morbidity and mortality increase as the serum albumin levels decrease, especially in patients where the level is less than 3.5g/dL.

RELATIONSHIP BETWEEN CRP AND SERUM ALBUMIN LEVELS

The body produces C-reactive protein (CRP) as a response to tissue trauma, infection, and inflammation. An elevation of more than 50mg/L is an accurate indicator of an acute inflammatory process in the dialysis patient. It may signal a retained failed allograft or a failed arteriovenous graft with undiagnosed infection. High CRP levels can be an indicator of mortality. CRP levels usually hit the highest level 2-3 days after an infection, increasing by as much as 100 times or more with a bacterial or viral infection. Within 1-2 weeks after the infection, the levels begin to drop. CRP values are useful in forecasting low serum albumin levels; evaluate any resistance to Epogen (epoetin alfa) therapy, evaluate the effectiveness of treatment of infections, and identify occult infections and chronic inflammation.

POTASSIUM

Potassium is necessary for the normal functioning of the neuromuscular, skeletal, and cardiac systems as well as smooth muscle activity and intracellular enzyme responses. It is the most prevalent intracellular positively charged ion (cation) and the second most plentiful in the body. Acid base balance affects potassium levels in the cells. Hypokalemia refers to an abnormally low level of serum potassium (less than 3.5mEq). Causes of hypokalemia include vomiting and diarrhea, abuse of laxatives, anorexia nervosa, diuretics, excessive perspiration, burns, and diet insufficiency. Symptoms appear as weakness, fatigue, and arrhythmias.

HYPERKALEMIA

When the serum potassium level reaches 5.5mEq/L, the condition is hyperkalemia. Excessive intake of potassium-rich foods is the usual culprit, but crush injury, transfusions, catabolic states, GI bleeding, hemolysis, and acidosis are also possible causes. The patient may complain of shortness of breath, cramping, diarrhea, dizziness, and muscle weakness. Cardiac effects range from arrhythmias to cardiac arrest. A rapid change in the serum potassium levels significantly affects the symptoms. Kayexalate, sodium bicarbonate, glucose, and insulin may be administered to treat this condition, but the most effective treatment is dialysis. Dialysis patients on digoxin must be closely monitored for toxicity as serum potassium decreases.

KIDNEY'S ROLE IN CALCIUM AND PHOSPHORUS HOMEOSTASIS

The kidney is instrumental in excreting excess phosphorus and producing the active form of vitamin D, called calcitriol. Calcitriol is a hormone which travels to the gut and aids in both phosphorus and calcium absorption. Moreover, calcium and phosphorus are regulated by the hormone PTH (parathyroid hormone). PTH is released from the parathyroid gland and functions to elevate serum calcium levels and lower phosphorus levels. Note that the kidneys are involved in both phosphorus excretion (under influence of PTH) and phosphorus absorption via calcitriol.

EFFECTS OF RENAL FAILURE ON CALCIUM AND PHOSPHORUS LEVELS

Renal failure causes a decrease in calcitriol production. Thus, there is lower calcium and phosphorus absorption taking place at the gut. The parathyroid gland senses the lower calcium levels and releases PTH. PTH attempts to raise calcium in the blood but also attempts to excrete excess phosphorus via the kidney. However, kidney function is subnormal and phosphorus is not excreted appropriately. The end result of renal failure is phosphorus accumulation and subnormal calcium levels. The reservoir for the body's calcium is bone. With PTH levels elevated to compensate for the lack of calcium absorption, bone disease ensues. The calcium is taken from bone and released into the bloodstream in response to PTH's stimulation. Interventions to bind phosphate in the gut and elevate serum calcium through oral vitamin D are needed in patients with chronic kidney disease.

ROLE OF PTH ON CALCIUM AND PHOSPHORUS

Parathyroid hormone (PTH) is stimulated by two mechanisms: either a low serum calcium level or elevated phosphorus. PTH acts to increase serum calcium and lower phosphorus. It increases calcium by two methods.

- The first is to stimulate the release of calcium from bone (the body's reservoir of calcium stores).
- The second is to stimulate the kidney to release calcitriol, the active form of Vitamin D. Calcitriol will raise serum calcium levels by increasing calcium absorption at the gut.

Finally, PTH acts to decrease serum phosphorus. It accomplishes this by acting on the kidneys to excrete phosphorus in the urine. In patients with chronic kidney disease, PTH is elevated because the kidneys do not respond appropriately. The kidneys can neither produce calcitriol nor excrete phosphorus. Thus, PTH levels rise (also known as secondary hyperparathyroidism) and a viscous cycle ensues.

IMPORTANCE OF CALCIUM-PHOSPHORUS PRODUCT

When the calcium and phosphorus levels reach a certain point, they can combine in the bloodstream and precipitate out. They form mineral deposits in organs as well as blood vessels, which is injurious to their function. Thus, nephrologists must keep track of the calcium-phosphorus product or simply multiply the serum calcium with the serum phosphorus. If the product exceeds 70, the patient is at increased risk of calcium-phosphorus deposition. Therefore, it is imperative to monitor the calcium-phosphorus product in all patients with chronic kidney disease with interventions to lower that product if necessary.

RENAL BONE DISEASE: RENAL OSTEODYSTROPHY

Renal osteodystrophy is a general term that includes many aspects of renal bone disease. It includes:

- Osteitis fibrosa cystica
- Osteomalacia
- Adynamic bone disease
- Mixed osteodystrophy

Briefly, osteitis fibrosa cystica exists when there is increased bone turnover from elevated PTH (hyperparathyroidism). Osteomalacia occurs when there is low bone turnover in combination with aluminum deposition. Adynamic bone disease occurs when bone turnover is low secondary to reduced parathyroid hormone. Finally, mixed osteodystrophy exists when there is a mixture of both high and low bone turnover. Again, renal osteodystrophy is a general term that encompasses all of the aforementioned entities.

OSTEITIS FIBROSA CYSTICA

Osteitis fibrosa cystica is the term used to define excess bone turnover in response to both elevated PTH (hyperparathyroidism) and low calcitriol. The driving force behind this response is elevated phosphorus levels and low calcium. The elevation in PTH causes calcium to be released from bone resulting in what is termed increased bone turnover. Increased bone turnover results in weakened bone structure and an osteoporosis of sorts. This leads towards an increased susceptibility to fractures (the most worrisome being hip fractures). Correction of increased bone turnover and thus osteitis fibrosa cystica is through administration of phosphate binders, consumption of low phosphorus diets, and supplementation of calcitriol.

OSTEOMALACIA

Osteomalacia is defined by low bone turnover secondary to aluminum deposition. In the past, efforts to decrease phosphorus were done with the use of aluminum binders. Aluminum was very good at binding phosphorus in the gut and thus preventing its absorption. Unfortunately, aluminum has some serious side effects. One side effect is that it deposits into bone and replaces the normal bony matrix. Thus, parathyroid hormone will act on bone, which is devoid of normal calcium and will be chronically elevated. This entity has largely vanished with the use of newer phosphate binders that do not use aluminum.

ADYNAMIC BONE DISEASE

Adynamic bone disease occurs when bone turnover is absent. The pathophysiology is as follows: parathyroid hormone levels are increased in response to low serum calcium and renal failure. Therapy is begun with calcium containing phosphate binders and calcitriol. The resulting increase in calcium and lowering of phosphorus causes PTH levels to decrease to near normal levels. This causes bone to be essentially dormant. The physiology of a patient with chronic kidney disease dictates that PTH levels at 1.5 – 2 times normal are needed in order to maintain healthy bone turnover. Otherwise, bone becomes dormant and essentially inactive. Thus, when treating patients for hyperphosphatemia and vitamin D deficiency, care must be taken not to be overzealous so as not to reduce PTH levels to normal.

EFFECTS OF METABOLIC ACIDOSIS ON NORMAL BONE HOMEOSTASIS

Metabolic acidosis contributes to renal bone disease by causing the release of calcium from bone. In patients with chronic kidney disease, amino acids are not readily excreted and the acids accumulate. The normal buffer for acids is bicarbonate. When the bicarbonate is exhausted, bone serves as a buffer. In acting as a buffer, bone releases calcium while absorbing the acids. Thus, bone is devoid of its vital elements making it weaker and more susceptible to fractures.

Correction of the acidosis will allow for the proper buffering of acids and allow calcium to remain in the bony matrix.

CALCIPHYLAXIS

Calciphylaxis is a rare complication of metastatic calcification. It occurs when the calcium-phosphorus product is high. Calcium precipitates in arteries and tissues including vital organs and skin. In contrast to metastatic calcification, calciphylaxis causes tissue ischemia. Patients frequently present with gangrenous skin that subsequently becomes infected. Treatment is primary prevention of an elevation of calcium-phosphorus product.

METASTATIC CALCIFICATION

Metastatic calcification occurs when calcium and phosphorus precipitate and deposit in blood vessels and tissues. This occurs when the calcium and phosphorus levels are high. High is defined by a calcium-phosphorus product of greater than 70. In order to prevent metastatic calcification, it is important to decrease serum phosphorus. This is accomplished with a diet restricted for phosphorus and judicious use of phosphate binders.

RENAL BONE DISEASE IN PEDIATRIC PATIENTS WITH CHRONIC KIDNEY DISEASE

Renal failure causes a metabolic acidosis. The acidosis causes displacement of calcium from the bones and retards bone growth. Hyperparathyroidism also retards bone growth. Thus, children with chronic kidney disease are of short stature. The biochemical changes along with malnutrition frequently leave children at the low end for height. Treatment of low stature includes correction of any nutritional deficiencies and chronic acidosis.

PROTEINURIA
MARKER OF KIDNEY DISEASE

Normal renal physiology allows for some protein to be filtered and excreted into the urine. By in large, most proteins are not filtered at the glomerulus and thus are never reabsorbed or excreted in the renal tubules. However, early marker of kidney damage is protein loss. There are different methods of urine collection but the most practical is a spot urinalysis. Spot refers to a one-time, random collection of urine during the day. The urine is sent for an albumin: creatinine ratio. If the ratio exceeds 30, there is evidence of early renal disease and modification of risk factors is important.

MEASUREMENT

Urinary protein is measured to assess renal damage. The most abundant protein in the serum is albumin. Albumin is normally not filtered nor secreted in the renal tubules. However, with renal damage, albumin is filtered and excreted in the urine. One method of measuring urinary protein is a 24-hour urine collection. The patient's urine is collected for 24 hours and is sent for albumin, creatinine and total protein. The major limitation for a 24-hour urine collection is difficulty in collecting urine over a prolonged period. Another method of measuring urinary protein is to collect a "spot" urine. The term spot refers to a random, one-time collection of urine. The advantage of a spot collection is that it is a one-time void, which is easier to collect. The urine is sent for an albumin:creatinine ratio. If the ratio is >30 mg/day than urinary protein is elevated and renal disease is present. Lastly, the routine urinalysis also measures proteinuria. However, it can only detect albumin levels of greater than 300 mg/day. Thus, it is not as sensitive as the albumin:creatinine ratio which can detect albumin levels as low as 30 mg/day.

PATHOPHYSIOLOGY OF ANEMIA OF CHRONIC KIDNEY DISEASE

The kidneys are important in releasing the hormone erythropoietin. Erythropoietin travels from the kidneys to the bone marrow and helps stimulate red blood cell formation. In patients with chronic kidney disease, there is nephronal loss. With less nephrons secreting adequate erythropoietin, there is less red blood cell production and hence anemia. To combat this, clinicians often give erythropoietin in patients with anemia. However, iron is also an important ingredient in red blood cell makeup. Therefore, by building iron stores in the body one can address the anemia in combination with erythropoietin if deemed necessary.

ANEMIA
ETIOLOGY, SYMPTOMS, AND EFFECT OF DIALYSIS

Anemia is a commonly found in uremic patients. Red blood cell production decreases in ESRD patients, and the cells that do form are frequently abnormal. Hematocrit values for a normal male are between 46 and 52%, and in a normal female, range from 40 to 45%. In the dialysis patient, the values are considerably lower with non-intervention patients leveling off in the 20-30% range. One cause of anemia in these patients is diminished erythropoietin (EPO), a hormone that stimulates the production of blood cells by bone marrow. Another is the inability to successfully absorb and use iron. In addition, the life span of the red blood cell decreases. Platelet abnormalities lead to bleeding from the gums, nose, GI tract, uterus, and skin. Symptoms of anemia include weakness, fatigue, and shortness of breath, chest pain, poor exercise tolerance, and inability to think clearly. During dialysis, the dialyzer may leak, frequent blood tests are done, and blood recovery may be incomplete. All of these are avoidable and care must be taken to reduce these causes of anemia.

PEDIATRIC PATIENTS WITH CHRONIC KIDNEY DISEASE

The pathophysiology of anemia in the pediatric population is similar to adults. However, the erythropoietin and iron requirements to correct the anemia are substantially higher. Erythropoietin should be administered subcutaneously. Supplemental iron needs to be administered both orally and, if needed, intravenously.

UREMIA
GI COMPLAINTS

Uremia is responsible for several GI complaints. Circulating uremic toxins cause nausea and vomiting in ESRD patients. The most frequent gastrointestinal complaints include the following:

- Nausea
- Poor appetite
- Metallic taste in mouth
- Vomiting
- Fetid breath (from decomposing urea)
- GI bleeding, often occult may be caused by platelet abnormalities and aggravated by the use of Heparin.
- Ammonia or hyperkalemia may cause diarrhea.
- Functional constipation and possible impactions may result from medications, diet, and lack of exercise or fluid restriction.

It is important to encourage patients to eat a high-fiber diet, exercise regularly, and if needed, use a stool softener.

NEUROLOGIC SYSTEM CHANGES

Neurologic symptoms may range from inattention to coma, depending upon the degree and cause of the uremic encephalopathy. Insomnia, restlessness, and anorexia are all seen when azotemia is present. Left unresolved, the symptoms could progress to emotional lability, lethargy, and vomiting. The most severe consequences of untreated azotemia can be coma and death. Commonly seen neurologic symptoms are anxiety, depression, agitation, and fatigue. Restless leg syndrome (RLS), in which the patient has uncontrollable urges to move the extremities when at rest, has been noted in uremia patients. Anemia and hyperphosphatemia may be contributing factors.

METABOLIC DISTURBANCES

Metabolism of glucose, lipids, and protein are often found to be abnormal in uremia patients. In nondiabetic ESRD patients, the decrease of cellular sensitivity to insulin results in abnormal glucose metabolism. In type 1 diabetes, hyperglycemic and hypoglycemic swings may be severe. Dialysis may decrease the insulin requirement. In type 2 diabetics, weight reduction, increased physical activity, and the administration of hypoglycemic agents may improve their glucose metabolism. Lipoprotein metabolism and structure are altered in ESRD patients. Type 4 hyperlipoproteinemia occurs regularly in this type of patient. Low levels of carnitine, a compound that is required for the transport of fatty acids into the mitochondria, may be found to play a part in this metabolic dysfunction. Protein metabolism dysfunction may result in wasting, impaired growth, and malnutrition. Poor intake, resulting in low serum albumin, depletion of nutrients during dialysis, and abnormal metabolism are all factors that influence this process. Loss of tissue mass may be obscured by edema.

Measuring Kidney Function

GFR

The best method for measuring kidney function and tracking the progression of chronic kidney disease is through the calculation of the glomerular filtration rate (GFR). The GFR is commonly estimated by two different equations: the Cockcroft-Gault equation and the modification of diet in renal disease (MDRD) equation.

COCKCROFT-GAULT EQUATION

The Cockcroft-Gault estimates the body's creatine clearance rate (*CC*, which itself is an estimate of GFR in mL/min) by the following:

$$CC = \frac{(140 - \text{age}) \times \text{body mass}}{72 \times \text{serum creatinine}}$$

Where *age* is in years, *body mass* is in kg, and *serum creatinine* is in mg/dL. For female patients, the result is multiplied by a factor of 0.85.

MDRD EQUATION

The MDRD estimates the body's GFR in mL/min by the following:

$$GFR = 186 \times \text{Serum Creatinine}^{-1.154} \times \text{Age}^{-0.203}$$

Or alternatively:

$$GFR = 170 \times \text{Serum Creatinine}^{-0.999} \times \text{Age}^{-0.176} \times \text{BUN}^{-0.17} \times \text{Albumin}^{0.318}$$

Where *age* is in years, *serum creatinine* and *BUN* are in mg/dL, and *Albumin* is in g/dL. For female patients, the result is multiplied by a factor of 0.742 (or 0.762 for the second equation). For African American patients, the result is multiplied by a factor of 1.21 (or 1.18 for the second equation).

COMPARING THE TWO METHODS

The Cockcroft-Gault equation is easily memorized and requires only one blood test to calculate. It also adjusts for the weight of the patient. However, its accuracy is questionable since it estimates a quantity which is itself an estimate of the quantity of interest.

The MDRD, although much more complicated, is the preferred equation because it is considered to be more accurate, particularly the alternate form of the equation. Unlike the CG, it does not account for patient weight, but it does account for ethnicity (sort of). It provides a modification only for African American patients.

The major limitation for both equations is that their accuracy falls off considerably at GFRs above 60. The equations are much more accurate for stages II – V. Both equations also rely heavily on having accurate lab results. Any significant amount of error in the lab results will render the estimates useless.

SCHWARTZ AND COUNAHAN-BARRATT EQUATIONS

The Schwartz equation is used to calculate the glomerular filtration rate in children. The equation is as follows: GFR = k x 0.55 x height (cm)/Creatinine (mg/dL), where k is a constant. The Counahan-Barratt equation is: GFR = k x 0.43 x height (cm)/Creatinine (mg/dL), where k is a constant. The major difference between the two equations is the constants (k). The equations use the proportional relationship between GFR and height and creatinine. Both equations lose some accuracy as glomerular filtration rates exceed 90 mg/min/1.73m^2.

LABORATORY TESTS NEEDED FOR PATIENTS WITH CHRONIC KIDNEY DISEASE

All patients with chronic kidney disease should be evaluated by a nephrologist. The evaluation should include the following blood work:

- Hemoglobin and hematocrit
- Iron studies
- Red blood cell indices (mean corpuscular volume and red cell distribution width)
- Electrolytes including phosphorus
- Urinalysis

The hemoglobin/hematocrit and red blood cell indices are important to evaluate those patients with anemia. Electrolyte measurements are used to adequately following the progression of CKD with estimation of glomerular filtration rates. It is also important to monitor phosphorus levels. Phosphorus is excreted by the kidney and in declining renal function, phosphorus accumulates. The urinalysis is important in evaluating proteinuria. However, the urinalysis is only effective at measuring heavy chain proteins, which are excreted at greater than 300 mg/dl. If less than 300 mg/dl of protein is excreted one can perform either a 24-hour urine collection for protein or a spot urine microalbumin/creatinine ratio. Less common tests ordered include erythropoietin levels and parathyroid hormone levels.

IMAGING MODALITIES TO DETECT UNDERLYING CAUSES OF CHRONIC KIDNEY DISEASE

The most common imaging modality used is the ultrasound. Renal ultrasounds reveal shape, size and contour of the kidneys. It can help identify hydronephrosis, cysts and tumors. Also, commonly used are CAT scans with/without intravenous contrast. Radiocontrast must be used with caution in patients with chronic kidney disease for it has been well documented to be nephrotoxic. However, cat scans provide a more precise image of the kidneys. Less commonly used imaging includes intravenous pyelograms, nuclear scans and MRI.

Decreased GFR Without Kidney Damage

Decreased glomerular filtration rate without kidney damaged is defined as a GFR between 60-89 mL/min/1.73m² without obvious signs of kidney failure. This is usually attributed to the aging process but can also be seen in young adults and children. The prognosis of decreased GFR is good and progression to stage V CKD is unlikely. Moreover, these patients may not present the sequale of chronic kidney disease including anemia and bone disease.

Preferred Method of Renal Replacement in Pediatric Patients

Nearly all pediatric patients with renal disease should be placed on the transplant list. While awaiting transplant the preferred method of renal replacement is peritoneal dialysis. Peritoneal dialysis affords the child freedom to attend school and live a more normal life. Hemodialysis is reserved for those patients when peritoneal dialysis is contraindicated or does not have the support structure.

Use of Dialyzers and Hemodialysis Machines in Pediatric Patients

The special use of dialyzers in children is aimed at the smaller body surface area. Hollow fiber dialyzers are the preferred dialyzer because of low compliance. The dialyzer surface area is also smaller to accommodate the smaller surface area. Dialyzer reuse is seldom used in pediatrics. Hemodialysis machines, however, do not differ from adult machines. Adult machines can be calibrated to adjust to pediatric volumes.

Complications

Aluminum in Patients with Chronic Kidney Disease

Major Sources of Aluminum

Previously, aluminum-based phosphate binders were commonly used and were a major source of aluminum toxicity. Aluminum helped bind phosphate in the gut. However, aluminum would also be absorbed and deposited into bones and cause dementia. Today, while aluminum-based phosphate binders are not readily used, other medicines may contain aluminum. These include the commonly used antacid aluminum hydroxide (trade name Maalox). Caution must be taken in using aluminum hydroxide in patients with chronic kidney disease. Overuse of antacids containing aluminum will lead to toxicity. Another source of aluminum is through the water system used for dialysis. Today, water purification systems have improved and water-testing methods are more sensitive today, preventing some causes of aluminum toxicity.

Toxicity

Aluminum is excreted by the kidneys. In patients with renal disease, the ability to excrete aluminum is hindered. Aluminum toxicity was a much larger problem when aluminum based phosphate binders were used. The aluminum would be absorbed by the gut and accumulate over time. Treatment of acute aluminum toxicity is via hemodialysis with a low aluminum dialysate concentration. Osteomalacia, dementia, anemia and hypercalcemia are products of chronic exposure to aluminum. Prevention of aluminum exposure is hugely important with avoidance of aluminum based phosphate binders and frequent monitoring of dialysis water system for elevated aluminum levels.

COMPLICATIONS: The major complications of aluminum toxicity include:

- Acute aluminum toxicity
- Dementia
- Hypercalcemia (by displacing calcium in bony matrix)

- Anemia
- Osteomalacia

Acute aluminum toxicity presents as an acute change in mental status. Patients need urgent and daily hemodialysis with low aluminum in the dialysate solution to remove the excess aluminum. Dementia is caused by chronic exposure to aluminum. The most common source of chronic aluminum exposure is a contaminated water system with high levels of aluminum. Chronic exposure to aluminum will also lead to osteomalacia (aluminum depositing in bone) and hypercalcemia (aluminum replacing calcium in bone).

Interventions

AIMS OF TREATMENT OF CHRONIC KIDNEY DISEASE

All patients with chronic kidney disease should have the following goals of treatment:

- Identify and treat comorbid conditions
- Diagnosis specific therapy
- Slowing the progression of chronic kidney disease
- Identifying and modifying cardiovascular risk factors
- Preparation for renal replacement therapy
- Renal replacement therapy if clinically indicated

MANAGEMENT NECESSARY IN TREATING EACH STAGE OF CHRONIC KIDNEY DISEASE

The management necessary in the treatment of each stage of chronic kidney disease is explained below:

- Stage I (GFR >90)—Diagnose and treat comorbid conditions, eliminate and/or treat known risk factors for chronic renal disease, slow the progression of cardiovascular disease, possible use of ace inhibitors or angiotensin receptor blockers.
- Stage II (GFR 60-89)—Estimate the progression of renal disease, eliminate and/or treat known risk factors for chronic renal disease, use ace inhibitors or angiotensin receptor blockers.
- Stage III (GFR 30-59)—Evaluate and treat complications of renal disease, use ace inhibitors or angiotensin receptor blockers.
- Stage IV (GFR 15-29)—Prepare for renal replacement therapy, use ace inhibitors or angiotensin receptor blockers if tolerated.
- Stage V (GFR <15)—Renal replacement via hemodialysis or peritoneal dialysis or transplant if uremia present.

INTERVENTIONS SHOWN TO INCREASE RATE OF DECLINE OF RENAL DISEASE

The following is a list of interventions which are currently recommend by the Kidney Disease Outcomes Quality Initiative (KDOQI):

- Strict glycemic control
- Blood pressure control to optimal levels
- Use of ace inhibitors or angiotensin receptor blockers
- Correction of anemia
- Management of hyperlipidemia
- Dietary protein restriction

All of the stated interventions help control the rate of decline of GFR and slows the progression towards end stage renal disease.

INITIAL ASSESSMENT OF CKD PATIENT

Initial assessment of the CKD patient should include the following:

- Comprehensive personal and familial history
- Complete physical examination
- Complete blood count
- Blood chemistry
- Complete urinalysis
- Renal ultrasound

GOALS OF COMPREHENSIVE ASSESSMENT

The goals of the comprehensive assessment are as follows:

- Distinguish between acute and chronic kidney disease
- Establish the etiology of the disease
- Determine the GFR
- Evaluate the rate of progression
- Analyze cardiovascular risk
- Assess protein excretion
- Gauge reversible damage
- Determine life style risks
- Evaluate dialysis vs. transplant
- Assess medications
- Determine complications of primary disease

FINAL DIAGNOSIS OF CKD DURING INITIAL ASSESSMENT OF PATIENT WITH KIDNEY DISEASE

The factors that influence the final diagnosis of CKD include the size of the kidney (determined by renal ultrasound), hemoglobin level, and ongoing assessment of renal function. In acute kidney disease, size is not a factor while in chronic disease, the evidence of small renal size in addition to the reduction of GFR for more than 3 months are indicative of chronic kidney disease. Assessing reversible renal dysfunction is an important step in determining chronic disease. Evaluation of extracellular fluid volume (ECFV), hypotension or extreme hypertension, cardiac failure, urinary obstruction, sepsis, and nephrotoxins is helpful in determining if damage could be reversible.

OPTIMAL BLOOD PRESSURES FOR PATIENTS WITH AND WITHOUT PROTEINURIA

According to the Joint National Committee for the prevention, detection, evaluation, and treatment of high blood pressure (JNC VI), the optimal blood pressure is a systolic of <120 and diastolic of <80. This is particularly relevant for those patients with proteinuria. Lowering blood pressure has been shown to dramatically reduce proteinuria and slow the progression of chronic kidney disease. However, in patients without documented proteinuria or risk factors for chronic kidney disease, acceptable blood pressures are systolic of <130 and diastolic of <85. The take home message is lower is better.

IMPORTANCE OF MANAGING HYPERTENSION

Hypertension can either cause or be a consequence of chronic kidney disease. It is a major public health risk and optimal management is important. Uncontrolled blood pressure can lead to coronary artery disease, stroke, kidney failure, left ventricular hypertrophy and congestive heart failure. The current guidelines advise that ace inhibitors be the agent of choice in managing hypertension. Multiple studies have found a decrease in mortality and morbidity in patients on ace inhibitors. Angiotensin receptor blockers are also acceptable alternatives to ace inhibitors.

Importance of Blood Pressure Management in Patients with Diabetes

Diabetes places patients at high risk for renal failure. Poor glycemic control causes renal damage and proteinuria. Up to 40% of patients with diabetes will progress to end stage renal disease and require dialysis. The concomitant presence of hypertension only exacerbates the risk and progression of chronic kidney disease. Therefore, it is imperative that patients with diabetes receive special attention in controlling both the serum glucose but also blood pressure. According to the Joint National committee for the prevention, detection, evaluation, and treatment of high blood pressure (JNC VI), the optimal blood pressure is 120/80. All diabetics should receive pharmacotherapy as well as diet and exercise regimens to achieve the stated goal. Again, the best agents in controlling blood pressure and reducing proteinuria are ace inhibitors. Angiotensin receptor blockers are excellent alternatives to ace inhibitors.

Pre-Dialysis Assessment

Pre-dialysis assessment is a very important step in preparing the patient for maintenance dialysis. Pre-dialysis assessments should include the following in order to best prepare a patient for maintenance dialysis:

- Afford suitable group and individualized predialysis education
- Assess social and psychological needs
- Determine home dialysis vs. hospital based treatment
- Decide on peritoneal dialysis vs. hemodialysis
- Rectify reversible factors precluding preferred dialysis mode
- Evaluate and treat infections (HIV, methicillin-resistant Staphylococcus aureus-MRSA, vancomycin-resistant Enterococcus-VRE, hepatitis B and C)
- Create dialysis access to permit optimal time for initiation
- Attain consent for ANZDATA (Australia and New Zealand Dialysis and Transplant Registry) compilation

Therapies in Addition to Dialysis

Dialysis alone cannot fully replace the function of a normal kidney. Supplemental therapies are extremely important in assuring the success of dialysis, these include the following:

- Suitable water and sodium intake for regulation of extracellular fluid volume (ECFV) and plasma osmolality
- Dietary restriction or supplementation for potassium balance
- Phosphate binders or vitamin D analogs (such as Calcitriol) when indicated for calcium/phosphate balance
- NaHCO3 for acid-base balance
- Avoidance of excess magnesium to maintain magnesium levels
- Calcitriol as needed for activation of 25-hydroxy cholecalciferol
- Angiotensin converting enzyme inhibitor (ACEI) or angiotensin receptor blocker (ARB) for the inhibition of the renin-angiotensin-aldosterone system.
- Erythropoietin, or similar, for synthesis of erythropoietin

Tracking Glomerular Filtration Rates

The rate of decline of kidney function increases in patients with chronic kidney disease. As the glomerular filtration rate decreases, the rate of decline towards dialysis also increases. Tracking the glomerular filtration rate aids clinicians in assessing how quickly renal function is declining. It also helps in assessing the effects of interventions on declining renal functions. Furthermore, as patients progress from stage to stage in chronic kidney disease, clinical interventions and management also change. For example, if a patient progresses from stage III to stage IV CKD, preparation must be made for renal replacement therapy. This includes both gaining access as well as preparing the patient and social support network for the emotional impact of dialysis.

IMPORTANCE OF TREATING CHRONIC KIDNEY DISEASE AS IT RELATES TO THE CARDIOVASCULAR SYSTEM

The leading cause of death in patients with renal failure is not renal related complications but rather coronary artery disease. Large epidemiological trials have clearly demonstrated that chronic kidney disease is an independent risk factor for coronary artery disease and cardiovascular related deaths. Renal failure is frequently associated with diabetes and hypertension (both known risk factors for cardiac disease). Glycemic control and treatment of high blood pressure are important risk modifiers of renal disease and cardiovascular deaths. Patients with chronic kidney disease should decrease salt intake, exercise and stop smoking. Furthermore, any elevations of cholesterol should be treated with diet, exercise and medications if necessary. Finally, ace inhibitors have been shown to be efficacious in slowing the progression of chronic kidney disease and in treating patients with heart failure. Ace inhibitors are also important in controlling blood pressure and have been shown to decrease cholesterol levels to some extent.

EVALUATING BONE METABOLISM

All patients with chronic kidney disease need the following blood tests in evaluating renal bone disease:

- Serum calcium
- Serum phosphorus
- Parathyroid hormone

The serum calcium is necessary to ensure that calcium levels are not dangerously low. Serum phosphorus is important to ensure that phosphorus levels are not high. Moreover, the product of serum calcium and phosphorus is important in determining a patient's risk for metastatic calcification. The calcium-phosphorus product should be kept below 70. Finally, the serum parathyroid hormone needs to be checked. In patients with chronic kidney disease, the PTH should be kept at about 1.5 – 2 times the upper limits of normal. Low PTH levels places patients at risk for adynamic bone disease. High PTH levels places patients at risk for osteoporosis and fractures.

RECOMMENDATIONS ON DIETARY PHOSPHORUS RESTRICTION

Most dietary phosphorus comes in the form of protein. Therefore, dietary protein restriction would greatly aid in lowering phosphorus intake. However, this only applies to patients with chronic kidney disease (CKD) Stages II-IV. In patients with stage V CKD, protein restriction is known to cause malnutrition. In fact, patients on dialysis frequently need more protein to ensure adequate nutrition. Thus, in patients with CKD Stages II-IV, protein restriction aids in lowering phosphorus. However, in patients with CKD Stage V, protein restriction is harmful. Therefore, CKD Stage V patients will require phosphate binders and elimination of dietary phosphorus from non-protein sources.

LIMITATIONS OF DIETARY CALCIUM INTAKE IN PATIENTS WITH ELEVATED PHOSPHORUS LEVELS

The limits of total daily calcium intake should not exceed 2000 mg. Furthermore, only 1500 mg of elemental calcium is permitted daily when given a calcium based phosphate binder. The rationale of limiting calcium intake is that excess calcium intake will result in increased calcium absorption. If too much calcium is absorbed, the calcium-phosphorus product may exceed the set limits of 70. A calcium-phosphorus product of greater than 70 leaves the patient susceptible to metastatic calcification and the rarer condition of calciphylaxis.

ANEMIA OF CHRONIC KIDNEY DISEASE

BENEFITS OF TREATMENT

Treating anemia of chronic kidney disease has both a survival and quality of life benefit.

- In patients on hemodialysis, treating anemia has led to overall survival. The mortality rates decreased overall in patients treated to appropriate hemoglobin levels.
- Other benefits include a reduction in left ventricular hypertrophy and decreased rates of hospitalizations.
- Moreover, the quality of life for patients improves. The exercise capacity is improved as measured by standardized six-minute walk tests.
- Overall, both survival and quality of life improved greatly with appropriate treatment of anemia.
- Conversely, not treating or under-treating anemia leads to increased mortality and decreased quality of life.

ACCEPTABLE HEMOGLOBIN LEVELS

According to the current National Kidney Foundation's Kidney Disease Outcomes Quality Initiative (KDOQI), acceptable hemoglobin levels for men and postmenopausal women is >12 and premenopausal women is >11. Why the disparity? The reasons are twofold:

- Men have more body mass and thus will require more hemoglobin
- Premenopausal women are still actively menstruating. The monthly blood loss will result in lower hemoglobin levels. This combined with low body masses allows for premenopausal women to have lower hemoglobin levels. Furthermore, postmenopausal women are no longer menstruating. Thus, they are held to the higher standard of >12. A hemoglobin level of under 12 would indicate a possibility of occult blood loss, namely colon cancer.

WORKUP

Anemia of chronic kidney disease is indicated in men and postmenopausal women with hemoglobin levels <12 and premenopausal women with hemoglobin levels <11. The workup should consist of the following blood test:

- Hemoglobin/hematocrit
- Red blood cell indices
- Iron studies
- Tsats (iron/total iron binding capacity x 100)
- Reticulocyte counts
- Occult fecal blood

A less common test includes serum erythropoietin. Low levels of erythropoietin in the absence of other causes of anemia suggest that failing kidneys are the cause of the anemia and appropriate supplementation is required.

GOALS OF THERAPY

The most basic goal is to achieve a hemoglobin level > 12 in men and postmenopausal women and > 11 in premenopausal women. However, achieving that goal is more complicated. Foremost, the body must have adequate iron stores. A lack of iron will lead to iron deficiency anemia and any further medicines, including erythropoietin will not be effective. Therefore, iron studies must be drawn. Ferritin levels (a measure of active iron) must be greater than 100. Another marker for iron stores is the iron/total iron binding capacity saturation percentage or Tsats. The appropriate Tsat level should exceed 20%. Anything less than 20% and iron must be replaced. Finally, erythropoietin levels should be drawn. If the level is low (often it is in patients with chronic kidney disease) then erythropoietin should be given to help correct the anemia. Remember, without the iron, erythropoietin is ineffective for it will stimulate red blood cells without the very important iron component needed.

Drawing Ferritin and Tsats

Ferritin is an indication of the amount of active iron stores in the body. Tsats stand for transferrin saturation percentage. It is derived by the following ratio: iron/total iron binding capacity multiplied by 100 to give a percentage. In formula form it is more commonly written as: Fe/TIBC x 100.

The Tsats are another indicator for iron stores in the body. Both the ferritin and Tsats will indicate if total body iron stores are low. If these markers for total body iron are indeed low, then one can assume the anemia is secondary to iron deficiency. Supplemental iron must be given. Furthermore, trending the ferritin and Tsats will aid the clinician in tracking response to therapy. The current guidelines stipulate that the ferritin should be >100 and Tsats >20%.

Drawing Hemoglobin/Hematocrit

The hemoglobin/hematocrit is the mainstay of documenting the presence of anemia and is necessary to follow progression of therapy. In order to diagnose anemia, the hemoglobin and hematocrit levels must be below the accepted lower limits of normal (<12 in men and postmenopausal women and <11 in premenopausal women). If the hemoglobin/hematocrit is below normal, then a work up of the type of anemia is necessary. It is important for clinicians to recognize that the anemia present is indeed secondary to chronic kidney disease and not another mechanism. Finally, trending hemoglobin/hematocrit levels is necessary to ensure appropriate responses to therapy.

Drawing Reticulocyte Counts

Reticulocytes are the precursors to mature red blood cells. They are released by the bone marrow and are indication of anemia if their levels are high. The physiological response to low hemoglobin/hematocrit is to stimulate the release of erythropoietin from the kidneys. Erythropoietin acts on the bone marrow to increase red cell production. The increase in red blood cell demand will cause an increase in reticulocyte production. If, however, the bone marrow is not functioning properly, the reticulocyte count will not respond appropriately to erythropoietin. Thus, in the presence of an anemia (low hemoglobin/hematocrit), a low reticulocyte count will indicate a bone marrow problem. In this instance a further workup is needed and supplemental iron and erythropoietin will not be effective.

Drawing Red Blood Cell Indices

The most important red blood cell index is the MCV or mean corpuscular volume. It is an indicator of how much hemoglobin and iron are within each red blood cell. If the hemoglobin and iron levels are low, the MCV will be low. However, excess hemoglobin or iron does not indicate a high MCV. A high MCV is usually found in patients with vitamin B12 and folate deficiencies. The other indices are also indicators of low iron or vitamin B12 and folate. This is just another measure to help clinicians narrow down the cause of the anemia. Again, a low MCV leads towards a diagnosis of iron deficiency anemia.

Examining Fecal Occult Blood

A frequent cause of anemia is the loss of blood via the gastrointestinal tract. Common causes of gastrointestinal blood loss include:

- Colon cancer
- Peptic and gastric ulcers
- Diverticulosis

The loss of blood will cause an anemia. In order to diagnose blood loss from the gastrointestinal tract, fecal hemoccult cards are used. The cards help identify blood loss which is not readily detectable with the naked eye. Blood loss via this route will help clinicians identify that the anemia is not necessarily due to chronic kidney disease and a further workup is need.

UPPER LIMITS OF ACCEPTABLE RANGES FOR TREATMENT

In men and postmenopausal women, the target hemoglobin is >12. In premenopausal women, the target hemoglobin is >11. However, iron supplementation can lead to adverse effects, chiefly cardiac, lung and liver dysfunction. In order to monitor iron therapy, the ferritin and Tsats are followed. Iron supplementation should be stopped if the ferritin exceeds 800 and the Tsat exceeds 50%. Again, higher levels than those stated are associated with iron overload states and can lead to cardiac, lung and liver dysfunction.

ADMINISTERING IRON

Iron is almost universally replenished orally. In fact, that is the preferred method. However, iron has some side effects, most notably constipation. Some patients may not be able to absorb iron because of gastrointestinal diseases including some malabsorption syndromes. Additionally, some patients do not adequately respond to oral iron therapy. Intravenous iron is the solution for those patients who cannot absorb iron or do not respond appropriately. Intravenous iron is administered during dialysis sessions with dosing according to their ferritin and Tsat levels.

PATIENT EDUCATION ABOUT STAGES OF ESRD

The chronic kidney disease patient should be educated about the stages of ESRD. Some of the benefits of pre-ESRD education are as follows:

- Decreases stress for patient and family members
- Improves the mortality and morbidity rates
- Increases self-care, aids in decision making
- Improves the ability to maintain employment
- Allows for informed decision making when replacement therapy is indicated

The American Association of Kidney Patients (AAKP) has created numerous programs to help those living with chronic kidney disease. Kidney Options is one such program that is co-sponsored by AAKP and Fresenius Medical Care North America. Informational materials are available on their website, through a newsletter, in brochures, and at local patient education venues. AAKP also works with Baxter Healthcare and the Stay in Touch program and provides educational mailings customized to the current needs of the patient as well as a toll-free hotline and a website.

DIET

The registered dietitian plays an important role in educating the ESRD patient. A proper diet may be beneficial by producing the following results:

- Delaying the need for dialysis
- Reducing the complications (phosphorus restriction to prevent bone complications)
- Providing adequate nutrition (improve morbidity and mortality)
- Improving the quality of life by customizing the diet (ethnic, lifestyle, variables)

Protein restriction, when implemented in concert with proper caloric intake, can be helpful in controlling uremic symptoms and in reducing the nitrogenous wastes. Kidney Disease Outcomes Quality Initiative (K/DOQI) recommends that patients with a GFR of less than 60mL/1.73m² should have their nutritional status, protein, and caloric intake assessed. When teaching the ESRD patient about proper diet, protein requirements play an important role. Areas that should be covered include the amount of protein that needs to be included in the daily intake. The latest research suggests 1.2 ± 0.2g/kg/day of protein with the higher range reserved for protein-malnourished patients. Half of the daily protein should come from high-biologic value protein (animal protein). The other half may be derived from certain fruits, vegetables, and grains. One cup of corn, potato, peas, pasta, or rice (cooked) contains approximately 4 grams of protein.

REVIEW OF MEDICATIONS

Every chronic kidney disease patient should have all medicines reviewed at each visit. According to the National Kidney Foundation, the following parameters should be reviewed:

- Dose adjustment based on glomerular filtration rate
- Detection of drug interactions
- Therapeutic drug monitoring
- Detection of adverse drug reactions on renal function

TREATING CONDITIONS COMMONLY FOUND IN ESRD PATIENT

Although there are no medications currently available to reverse or cure kidney failure, several drugs have proven valuable in treating conditions commonly found in the ESRD patient. Drugs administered in CKD patients include the following:

- Cinacalcet HCl (Senispar) is a drug used for lowering the level of parathyroid hormone (PTH) in the blood. CKD interferes with metabolism of calcium, phosphate, and vitamin D. CKD leads to a condition known as hyperparathyroidism in which elevated levels of PTH if left untreated may lead to uremic bone disease. This is an oral medication. Possible side effects associated with Senispar are nausea, vomiting, and transient low blood calcium levels.
- Furosemide (Lasix) and bumetanide (Bumex) are commonly used diuretics. They are available in oral form and as injections. Side effects may include dizziness, dry mouth, frequent urination, and weakness.

OVER THE COUNTER MEDICATIONS FOR ESRD PATIENTS

Over the counter medications may be ordered for the ESRD patient. Over-the-counter medications that may be prescribed for the ESRD patient include the following:

- Sodium Bicarbonate is often used for treatment of metabolic acidosis, a condition that occurs due to the damaged kidney's inability to synthesize ammonia and excrete hydrogen ions. It is administered orally when taken as an over-the-counter medication. Sodium levels must be monitored when this medication is taken.
- Calcium Carbonate and Calcium Acetate are oral medications that are used to bind phosphate for preventing bone loss due to abnormally high phosphate levels in the blood. Side effects may include constipation, slow heart rate, and loss of appetite.

HYPERTENSION

According to the Seventh Report of the Joint National Committee on Prevention, Detection, Evaluation, and Treatment of High Blood Pressure (JNC 7), hypertension is divided in to the following stages:

Stage	Blood Pressure Range
Normal	<120/<80 mmHg
Prehypertension	120-139/80-89 mmHg

Stage	Blood Pressure Range
Stage 1	140-159/90-99 mmHg
Stage 2	>160/>100 mmHg

ANTIHYPERTENSIVE MEDICATIONS

The most common medications include:

- Thiazide diuretics—Block sodium and chloride at the distal convoluted tubule resulting in excess water excretion
- Beta blockers—Act on B1 receptors on the heart to slow heart rate and thus, cardiac output
- Ace-Inhibitors—Act by blocking angiotensin converting enzyme which is crucial to the conversion of angiotensin I to angiotensin II (potent vasoconstrictor)
- Angiotensin Receptor Blockers—Block the angiotensin II receptors
- Calcium channel blockers—Slow the heart rate as well as vasodilate the peripheral circulation

TREATMENT OF HYPERPARATHYROIDISM

Two medications prescribed for the treatment of hyperparathyroidism are as follows:

- Paricalcitol (Zemplar) injection is an aggressive treatment for secondary hyperparathyroidism. The usual administration route for paricalcitol (Zemplar) is intravenous. This medication decreases the PTH levels and has a negligible effect on phosphorus and calcium. Digitalis toxicity must be monitored if hypercalcemia is present. Paricalcitol is contraindicated in patients with vitamin D toxicity and hypercalcemia.
- Doxercalciferol (Hectorol) is also used to control PTH and hyperparathyroidism. It may be administered intravenously or orally. The patient needs to be monitored for hypercalcemia, hyperphosphatemia, and hypoparathyroidism while on Hectorol.

ACE INHIBITORS

Chronic kidney disease is frequently accompanied by protein loss in the urine. The inability of the kidneys to retain protein is not only an indication of renal failure but is injurious to the nephron. Proteins are harmful to the kidney and measures to slow protein filtration and loss is important to prevent kidney disease progression. Ace inhibitors act by decreasing the amount of protein loss in the kidney. They do so by blocking the actions of the angiotensin-converting enzyme. This enzyme helps release angiotensin II, which is a potent vasoconstrictor. By blocking this enzyme, the renal arteries (particularly the efferent arteriole) are allowed to vasodilate. The vasodilatory effects of ace inhibitors slow the amount of protein being delivered and filtered at the kidneys. Thus, protein loss is curbed and progression of chronic kidney disease delayed.

PHOSPHATE BINDERS

There are three main categories of phosphate binders:

- Aluminum based
- Calcium based
- Non-calcium based

Aluminum based phosphate binders were used to bind phosphate in the gut and prevent its absorption. However, significant side effects of aluminum including osteomalacia and dementia have eliminated aluminum as a viable option. Calcium based phosphate binders are the most commonly used. They bind phosphorus in the gut with some absorption of elemental calcium. The main side effect of calcium-based binders is hypercalcemia. Finally, non-calcium-based binders are new to the market and are increasingly popular. They are polymers that bind to intestinal phosphorus and have few side effects in contrast to aluminum and calcium-based binders.

Phosphorus levels should be kept at normal to high normal levels in patients with chronic kidney disease. Dietary restriction should be the first attempt at reducing phosphorus levels. However, in patients with persistently elevated phosphorus despite dietary restriction, phosphate binders should be used. In patients with chronic kidney disease stages III – IV, calcium-based binders are the first choice. Calcium based binders are preferred in this patient population for the supplemental calcium will aid in preserving bone integrity and reducing PTH levels. However, in patients with stage V CKD, either calcium based or non-calcium-based binders are preferred. The difference is that in patients with stage V CKD, they often have higher phosphorus levels. Any supplemental calcium absorbed with calcium-based binders may precipitate metastatic calcification. Therefore, non-calcium-based binders are equally as effective in patients with stage V CKD.

Management of Hypercalcemia in Patients with Chronic Kidney Disease Stage V

In patients on renal replacement therapy and with a serum calcium level above 10.2 the following measures should be taken to reduce serum calcium. First, in patients taking calcium-based phosphate binders the dose should be reduced. If that does not work, the alternative of using a non-calcium-based binder should be implemented. Second, in patients taking supplemental vitamin D the dose should be reduced or eliminated. Finally, if the aforementioned steps did not adequately reduce serum calcium levels then using a lower calcium dialysate solution should be used. Hopefully, dialysate solutions with lower calcium levels will help eliminate excess serum calcium with each dialysis session.

Vitamin D Supplementation

Patients with chronic kidney disease are subject to hyperparathyroidism. In order to maintain parathyroid hormone levels at acceptable levels, the serum calcium and phosphorus must be at near normal levels. Moreover, a deficiency of vitamin D will lead to excess release of PTH. Thus, in patients with PTH levels above acceptable limits as determined by the stage of chronic kidney disease a vitamin D level must be checked. If the vitamin D level is below normal, supplemental vitamin D should be offered. Hopefully, the vitamin D will lower PTH levels to acceptable levels (1.5 – 2 times normal). Serial vitamin D and PTH levels along with serum calcium and phosphorus need to be checked to monitor therapy.

Limitations in Patients with Chronic Kidney Disease

Patients with chronic kidney disease and elevated PTH levels with concomitant low vitamin D stores will need vitamin D supplementation. Vitamin D is administered in oral form and it will increase absorption of calcium and phosphorus. Yet, caution must be taken so as not to raise the serum calcium and phosphorus levels to above acceptable limits. If the serum calcium becomes elevated, a lower dosage or discontinuation of vitamin D is indicated. If the serum phosphorus becomes elevated, addition of a phosphate binder or discontinuation of vitamin D is indicated.

Hypocalcemia

In patients with low serum calcium levels care must be taken to ensure that the patient is not symptomatic. Signs of low calcium include tetany, bronchospasm, muscle twitching, and most severely seizures. Supplemental calcium should come in the form of oral calcium salts and vitamin D. Again, caution must be taken in supplementing calcium. Overzealous calcium supplementation could result in hypercalcemia and precipitate calcium deposition in tissues and vessels.

Erythropoietin

Side Effects

The most common side effects of erythropoietin include the following:

- Hypertension
- Seizures
- Increased clotting and hyperkalemia

As erythropoietin takes effect some patients will see an elevation of their blood pressure. Proper monitoring and increasing antihypertensive medicines may be necessary in some patients. While increases in seizure activity, clotting and hyperkalemia have been reported, there is no need to more closely monitor patients for these side effects. Furthermore, there are no recommended prophylactic measures necessary to prevent the onset of seizures or clotting. There is no role for antiepileptic or anticoagulation prophylactically in patients on erythropoietin.

Monitoring of Hemoglobin Levels

According to the national kidney foundation, the hemoglobin and hematocrit levels should be monitored every 1 to 2 weeks following the initiation of erythropoietin. The erythropoietin dose should be given until a stable hemoglobin level is reached. If the hemoglobin is below the stated goals of >12 in men and postmenopausal women and >11 in premenopausal women, then a higher dose of erythropoietin should be given. The cycle of dose adjustments and monitoring should be continued until the target is achieved. Once the target is achieved, hemoglobin can be monitored every 2-4 weeks.

Delivering Erythropoietin

Erythropoietin is most effective when administered via the subcutaneous route. It can also be given intravenously. While most studies of erythropoietin have been through the intravenous route, subcutaneous is the preferred method. Foremost, it achieves higher levels of hemoglobin than the intravenous route, is less expensive and less dosing is required. The one major drawback to subcutaneous administration is the discomfort to the patient and the frequent changing of skin sites with each dose. Erythropoietin is administered based on dry weight and can be given with each dialysis session or once monthly depending on the manufacturer.

<u>Alternatives to Subcutaneous Injections:</u> If a patient does not tolerate subcutaneous administration of erythropoietin, the alternative would be intravenous. Intravenous erythropoietin is less effective in raising the hemoglobin/hematocrit level and is more expensive. However, it is the best alternate to subcutaneous injections. The dose of intravenous erythropoietin should be increased by 50% as compared to subcutaneous dosing. In hemodialysis patients, the intravenous form should be given through either the arterial or venous port. The intravenous forms are given once per week in contrast to the three times per week subcutaneous method.

Maintaining Patient Compliance with Subcutaneous Erythropoietin Injections

The best method of maintaining patient compliance is through patient education. It is important for all patients to understand the importance of treating anemia, but also to take erythropoietin subcutaneously. The subcutaneous delivery to erythropoietin has been shown to increase the hemoglobin/hematocrit response more effectively and is less expensive. Another method for increasing compliance is to rotate injection sites so as to minimize local irritation. One should also use the smallest possible gauge needle (usually 29). Moreover, using a multi-dose preparation containing benzyl alcohol will help compliance. Benzyl alcohol acts as a local anesthetic, which helps minimize any pain. Finally, encourage the patients to self-administer the injections. This will help empower the patient and allow them to take control over their therapy.

LIMITATIONS OF GIVING ERYTHROPOIETIN INTRAVENOUSLY

Intravenous erythropoietin should be avoided for the following reasons:

- It is less effective than subcutaneous regimens in raising the hemoglobin/hematocrit level.
- It is more expensive.
- It requires intravenous access.

Studies have clearly demonstrated that the subcutaneous route of erythropoietin is more effective in treating anemia than the intravenous method. Furthermore, intravenous erythropoietin is far more expensive and will pose deterrence to both dialysis facilities and patients. Finally, in patients on peritoneal dialysis and those with chronic kidney disease stages II – IV, the need to obtain intravenous access is very cumbersome. Most patients will not want a needle stick every week to receive their erythropoietin dose. In hemodialysis patients, the erythropoietin can be given via either the arterial or venous lines at any point during the session.

ERYTHROPOIETIN TREATMENT FAILURE

The most common cause of erythropoietin treatment failure is iron deficiency. Adequate iron stores are necessary to ensure erythropoietin's efficacy. Less common causes include:

- Infection and inflammation
- Chronic blood loss
- Osteitis fibrosa
- Aluminum toxicity
- Hemoglobinopathies
- Folate or vitamin B12 deficiency
- Multiple myeloma
- Malnutrition
- Hemolysis

The underlying conditions should be treated to ensure adequate responses to erythropoietin. In cases where erythropoietin therapy is refractory, patients with anemia should be transfused with packed red blood cells.

CHRONIC BLOOD LOSS: Chronic blood loss always leads to iron deficiency. Any mechanism that causes iron deficiency will lead to erythropoietin treatment failure. The most common causes of chronic blood loss include:

- Gastrointestinal blood loss
- Menstruation
- Frequent blood draws in hemodialysis patients

Gastrointestinal blood loss is usually due to:

- Colorectal cancer
- Diverticulosis
- Peptic and gastric ulcers

Premenopausal women are always at increased risk for iron deficiency anemia because of menstruation. Hemodialysis patients frequently have their blood taken before and after each dialysis session. The chronic phlebotomy leads to iron losses and depletion of total body iron stores. All patients with chronic blood loss will frequently need iron supplementation.

<u>INFECTION/INFLAMMATION</u>: Chronic infections and inflammatory states have been well documented as causes of erythropoietin treatment failure. The most common causes of infections include:

- Vascular access site infections
- Chronic osteomyelitis
- Human immunodeficiency virus

The most common chronic inflammatory states include surgical patients and patients with chronic rheumatological conditions. Treatment of the underlying condition is instrumental in resolving erythropoietin treatment failure. The mechanism of infectious/inflammatory states as causing erythropoietin failure is poorly understood.

<u>ALUMINUM TOXICITY</u>: Aluminum toxicity occurs when patients with chronic kidney disease take certain phosphate binders. Older phosphate binders used to contain aluminum, which helped bind phosphorus in the gastrointestinal tract and limit its absorption. The use of aluminum can build in patients and deposit in bone. Bony deposition of aluminum can lead to bone marrow failure and thus resistance to erythropoietin.

<u>OSTEITIS FIBROSA</u>: Osteitis fibrosa is found in many patients with chronic kidney disease. In response to phosphorus retention, parathyroid hormone levels increase. Parathyroid hormone functions to lower serum phosphorus while concomitantly increasing serum calcium. The major body store for calcium is bone. The increase in parathyroid hormone causes increased bone turnover. The increase in bone turnover also affects the makeup of bone marrow (the place where red blood cell production takes place). Increased bone activity leads to fibrosis of the bone marrow. With fibrosis of the bone marrow, there is no room for erythropoietin's ability to stimulate red blood cell production.

FOLATE OR VITAMIN B12 DEFICIENCY

Folate and vitamin B12 are also essential for proper hemoglobin synthesis. A deficiency in either one will result in a macrocytic anemia. Anemia caused by folate or b12 deficiency must be corrected. While there is no direct correlation between folate and b12 and erythropoietin's mechanism of action, a macrocytic anemia must first be corrected prior to seeing any response to erythropoietin. Erythropoietin increases red blood cell production, but will not be effective if vital elements (folate and b12) for hemoglobin synthesis are missing.

<u>HEMOGLOBINOPATHIES:</u> The most common hemoglobinopathy encountered is sickle cell disease. Sickle cell disease is a condition where hemoglobin does not function normally. This leads to a loss of oxygen carrying capacity. Erythropoietin will increase bone marrow production of defective red blood cells. The red blood cells produced will not transport oxygen effectively, rendering erythropoietin relatively ineffective. Other less common causes of hemoglobinopathies include alpha and beta thalassemia, most commonly found in persons of Asian descent.

<u>MALNUTRITION</u>: Many patients with chronic kidney disease, particularly patients on hemodialysis are frequently malnourished. Malnutrition is associated with the loss of essential and nonessential vitamins and minerals. The lack of nutrition will presumably not provide the required elements in hemoglobin and red blood cell production. This will, of course, render erythropoietin ineffective. The bone marrow will not respond appropriately if the essential requirements for red blood cell synthesis are not present.

<u>HEMOLYSIS</u>: Hemolysis is frequently found when dialysate solutions are contaminated and kinks in the lines are found. Hemolysis causes acute red blood cell destruction. Erythropoietin will stimulate the bone marrow to produce red blood cells. Yet, newly formed red blood cells are destroyed, and will serve

no purpose. It is important that the cause of the hemolysis is found and treated prior to initiating treatment with erythropoietin.

Administering Iron Along with Erythropoietin

Erythropoietin stimulates the bone marrow to produce red blood cells. Red blood cells are largely made of hemoglobin, the protein necessary for oxygen transport. The main component of hemoglobin is iron. Iron is instrumental in hemoglobin's ability to carry oxygen from the lungs to the tissues. If erythropoietin stimulates red blood cell production, the body must be prepared to accommodate the increase in demand. The most important body store in this instance will be iron. If the body is does not have adequate iron stores, erythropoietin will essentially be ineffective. This is because erythropoietin will stimulate red blood cells without their most important ingredient: iron.

Erythropoietin Therapy Without Iron Supplementation

As long as anemia persists, erythropoietin is indicated. Furthermore, erythropoietin is indicated as maintenance therapy to maintain appropriate hemoglobin levels. But iron is only indicated if iron stores are below normal. Iron supplementation should continue until body stores are completely replenished. Caution must be taken with iron supplementation so as not to cause an iron overload state. Finally, hemodialysis patients frequently provide blood samples before and after each dialysis session. This phlebotomy leaves them in a chronic iron deficiency state. Therefore, it is frequently common to find hemodialysis patients taking both erythropoietin and iron as maintenance therapy.

Health Care Team Members

The following are members of the health care team who support patients with chronic kidney disease:

- Nephrologist: This is a physician who is specialized in kidney-related diseases.
- Advanced Practitioner: This is a Physician Assistant (PA) or Nurse Practitioner (NP). These providers work closely with the Nephrologist in providing medical care.
- Nephrology Nurse: This is a Registered Nurse who has undergone additional training and certification to provide care to patients with chronic kidney disease.
- Renal Nutritionist: This is a dietitian who has undergone certification to help meet the nutritional needs of patients with chronic kidney disease.
- Nephrology Social Worker: This professional is a licensed or certified social worker who helps kidney patients and their families obtain the help they need at home. They also coordinate services provided by community agencies to help patients when they are home.
- Renal Technologist: This person works under the nurse and is often the person most directly involved with the patient during dialysis treatments. They often start and end the treatment and monitor the patient throughout.
- Financial Counselor: This person helps the patient and family with questions regarding insurance coverage and patient responsibility for any services provided.

Early Referral of ESRD Patient to Nephrologist

Early referral of the ESRD patient to a nephrologist has been shown to decrease the mortality rate for the ESRD patient. Some of the benefits of early referral of the ESRD patient to a nephrologist include the following:

- Establishment of dietary prescription
- Placement of peritoneal or vascular access
- Timely diagnosis and treatment of hypertension, anemia, phosphatemia, and acidosis

MANAGING LATER STAGES OF CKD

The tasks associated with managing the later stages of CKD include preparing the patient for dialysis, determining the best mode of dialysis (outpatient hemodialysis center, peritoneal dialysis, or home hemodialysis) dietary evaluation with phosphorus and volume management, and administration of necessary immunizations. A decision must be made to determine the best course of treatment: either chronic dialysis or renal transplantation.

EMOTIONAL IMPACT ON PATIENTS WITH CHRONIC KIDNEY DISEASE

Chronic kidney disease, particularly dialysis, has a huge emotional and social impact on patients. Patients on dialysis lose a lot of freedom and their quality of life decreases. It has been widely reported that patients with chronic kidney disease have a higher incidence of depression. It is important that a social support network be intimately involved in the care of all patients with chronic kidney disease. Social workers are extremely important in coordinating home services and addressing family and social issues with all patients.

STRESS

Psychosocial aspects that affect the ESRD patient are often associated with stress. Psychosocial issues affect the general health of the ESRD patient. Stress associated with ESRD and dialysis comes from many factors and may have a significant effect on the overall outcome of the treatment. Depression, that may be the result of chronic illness, and a lack of social support have been linked to mortality in numerous studies of ESRD patients. Several of the stressors that affect the ESRD patient include the following:

- Effects of the illness
- Family dynamics
- Dietary restrictions
- Time constraints
- Financial responsibilities
- Functional restraints
- Employment adjustments
- Sexual changes
- Staff interactions
- Personal role modification
- Medication effects
- Concerns regarding life span

NATIONAL KIDNEY FOUNDATION

The National Kidney Foundation, Inc. is the major health organization that has established guidelines in the care of patients with kidney diseases. Specifically, the National Kidney Foundation has established the kidney disease outcomes quality initiative (KDOQI). KDOQI provides evidence-based guidelines to all clinicians caring for patients with renal disease. The guidelines include managing anemia in chronic kidney disease, bone metabolism in chronic kidney disease, hemodialysis, peritoneal dialysis, vascular access, nutrition, dyslipidemias, hypertension and antihypertensive therapy, cardiovascular disease in dialysis patients and pediatric bone.

Hemodialysis

METRIC SYSTEM ABBREVIATIONS

The following are the major abbreviations for the metric system, assuming grams is the unit measure:

$$\text{kilo (kg)} - 1000 = 10^3$$
$$\text{deka (Dg)} - 10 = 10^1$$
$$\text{deci (dg)} - 1/10 = 10^{-1}$$
$$\text{centi (cg)} - 1/100 = 10^{-2}$$
$$\text{milli (mg)} - 1/1000 = 10^{-3}$$
$$\text{micro (µg)} - 1/1000000 = 10^{-6}$$
$$\text{nano (ng)} - 1/1000000000 = 10^{-9}$$

ELEMENT

Elements are the most fundamental substances in nature. They cannot be broken down into further components without changing their essential properties. They are made up of atoms, which share the same proton number. For example, helium is composed of two protons and exists as a gas naturally. However, if one were to take one proton away from helium, then it would no longer be helium. It would now exist as hydrogen, which is a totally different gas with different properties altogether.

ATOM

An atom is the smallest particle of an element that still retains the properties of that element. Atoms are composed of a central nucleus comprised of protons and neutrons with surrounding electrons. The number of protons defines what type of atom it is, e.g. hydrogen has one proton and helium has two protons. Protons have a positive charge and a much larger in comparison to electrons, which have a negative charge. Neutrons are also large particles but they possess neither a positive or negative charge.

COMPOUND

A compound is a combination of different elements. For example, 2 parts hydrogen and one-part oxygen comprise a compound. In contrast, hydrogen and oxygen alone are simply elements. Separately they exist as gases. However, in combination they form water. Compounds can be organic (containing a carbon atom, and most also containing a hydrogen atom) or inorganic (generally NOT containing a carbon atom). A few inorganic compounds do contain carbon, such as carbon monoxide, carbon dioxide and sodium bicarbonate.

SOLUTION

A solution is a mixture of dissolved particle (solute) into a liquid (solvent). Each solution has different properties based on the solute and solvents used. For example, salt water can be thought of a solution. Sodium Chloride (NaCl) is dissolved in water (H_2O) to form salt water. Be careful not to confuse solutions with compounds. NaCl is one compound and H_2O is another compound. They both retain their properties and the mixture (salt water) does not make a new compound. Understanding solutions is important, particularly with dialysate composition.

CONCENTRATION

Concentration is defined as the amount of solute divided by the amount of solvent usually expressed as gm/L. For example, dissolving 1 gram of salt into one liter of water will yield a concentration of 1gm/L. Dissolving 10 grams of salt into one liter of water will yield a concentration of 10gm/L. Intuitively, one can deduce that the latter is more concentrated than the former and thus would taste saltier. Concentrations are important when comprising dialysate solutions and examining blood levels as well.

ION

An ion is a particle capable of carrying an electric charge. Ions are subdivided according to charge:

- A positively charged ion is called a cation.
- A negatively charged ion is called an anion.

It is also important to remember that ions can be either elements like sodium, which carries a positive charge or compounds like bicarbonate (HCO_3), which carries a negative charge.

ELECTROLYTES

An electrolyte is a substance that dissolves in water to form ions. Ions are particles that carry an electric charge. The most often measured electrolytes include:

- Sodium (Na)
- Potassium (k)
- Chloride (Cl)
- Calcium (Ca)
- Magnesium (Mg)

It is also important to remember that sodium and potassium carry one positive charge (cation). Calcium and magnesium carry two positive charges (cations). Chloride, however, carries one negative charge (anion).

SEMIPERMEABLE

Semipermeable means allowing the passage of some things while restricting others. For example, dialysis filters are considered semipermeable. That is because they are filters with holes that only permit the passage of certain sized molecules (usually <500 Daltons). Any molecule with a size of greater than 500 Daltons cannot pass through the dialysis filter. Thus, dialysis membranes filter very small molecules such as urea and electrolytes very well. They remove urea from the blood but not more vital elements such as albumin and other proteins.

OSMOSIS

Osmosis is the movement of fluids from an area of low concentration to an area of high concentration. For example, suppose we place two fluids in the same container separated by a membrane that only allows the passage of fluids. One solution will contain a concentration of 10mg/L of salt (NaCl). The other solution will contain a concentration of 1 mg/L of salt (NaCl). Remember, only fluid is allowed to pass from one part of the container through the membrane (not particles). Because the fluid is more concentrated on the 10mg/L side, fluid will shift from the 1 mg/L side towards the 10mg/L side. Fluid will continue to move until the concentrations on both sides are equal. Another way of looking at it is that there is more fluid on the 1 mg/L side and it will, via osmosis, travel down its concentration gradient towards the 10mg/L.

DIFFUSION

Diffusion is similar conceptually to osmosis. Osmosis is the movement of *fluids* from an area of low concentration to an area of high concentration, while diffusion is the movement of *particles* from an area of high concentration to low concentration. For example, suppose again that we place two fluids in the same container separated by a membrane that only allows the passage of particles, rather than fluids.

One solution will contain a concentration of 10mg/L of salt (NaCl). The other solution will contain a concentration of 1 mg/L of salt (NaCl). Remember, only particles are allowed to pass from one part of the container through the membrane (not fluid). Because the fluid is more concentrated on the 10mg/L side, *particles* will shift down their concentration gradient towards the 1 mg/L side. Particles will continue to move until the concentrations on both sides of the membrane are equal.

DISTRIBUTION OF WATER IN THE HUMAN BODY

Total body water can be easily quantified by multiplying body weight by 60%. Thus, the human body is 60% water weight. Yet, how that water is distributed can be subdivided into the following compartments:

- Intravascular
- Interstitial
- Intracellular

Intravascular refers to the water content found in arteries and veins. Interstitial refers to the water content found in capillaries and organs. Intracellular refers to the water content inside the cell only. Most body water is located intracellularly with less in the interstitium and least in the vascular space. Patients with chronic kidney disease may not generate enough urine and thus water balance is disturbed. Hemodialysis patients frequently need excess water removed at each session and the post dialysis weight is commonly referred to as dry weight (weight after dialysis where excess fluid is removed).

WATER HOMEOSTASIS IN THE AVERAGE ADULT

The most important principle in water balance is to understand that a normal adult will take in as much water as he/she will lose. If one takes in excess water, there will be a net positive water balance. If one loses more water, there will be a net negative water balance. The average adult takes in water from ingestion of solids and liquids and from oxidative processes in the body. The total is roughly about 2500 ml. Water is lost through feces, urine and insensible loss. Insensible loss describes water lost via the skin (to cool the body) and via the lungs (with each expiration). If, for example, one exercises, insensible loss via the skin will increase. In order to maintain water balance, the body will trigger thirst sensors and obligate one to drink water. Conversely, if one drinks excess water then one will urinate more to maintain water balance.

CAUSES OF HYPOTENSION

Hypotension is most commonly caused by excess water volume removal, antihypertensive medications and acute infections causing sepsis and arrhythmias. Less common causes of hypotension include anaphylaxis, liver cirrhosis and improper blood pressure measurements. In order to differentiate the cause of hypotension, a complete history and physical should be performed prior to any new dialysis patient begins chronic dialysis. Furthermore, any new changes in medical conditions or medications should be duly noted. The sepsis syndrome would be associated with fevers, high white blood cell count and a source of infection (usually access site). Arrhythmias should be suspected if the electrolytes are abnormal and if the pulse rate changes abruptly. Changes in antihypertensive medication dosages frequently lead to hypotension. Anaphylaxis occurs when a severe allergic reaction occurs to a particular food, latex or medicines. Most commonly, an antibiotic is given during dialysis and seconds later the patient is hypotensive. Other signs of an allergic reaction include fevers, hives, and itching. Liver cirrhosis is suggested by history. Poorly measured blood pressures are frequently found with inappropriate cuff sizes, improper placement of the cuff and with automated blood pressure machines.

pH

pH is defined as the negative log of hydrogen ion concentration. It is an indication of the acidity or alkalinity of a solution. The equation is rarely used to compute pH in everyday use but the values are important. Water has a pH of 7.0, which is considered neither an acid nor base. The lower the pH the more acidic a solution becomes. Conversely, the higher the pH the more basic a solution is. The range of acidic levels is between 1.0 – 6.99 and the range for basic solutions is between 7.01 to 14.0. Normal serum pH ranges between 7.35 – 7.45. Understanding pH values is important as it relates to patients with chronic kidney disease. The kidneys are important in filtering and excreting waste. When the waste products accumulate, a total body acidosis ensues. Acidosis is commonly found in patients with chronic kidney disease.

Normal Blood Flow to Kidneys

The kidneys are unique in that 25% of total blood flows from the heart supply the kidneys exclusively. Blood reaches the kidneys through the renal artery. The renal artery then divides into smaller branches until they reach the afferent arteriole. Afferent means carrying towards. The afferent arteriole leads towards the glomerulus, the apparatus where blood is filtered and toxins removed. After the glomerulus, the efferent arteriole carries blood away from the kidneys toward the renal veins (efferent means to carry away). The renal veins carry the blood back towards the heart where the cycle is repeated. The site of action of ace inhibitors is at the efferent arteriole. Be careful not to confuse normal renal blood flow with urine formation. Urine formation is a completely separate process.

Formation of Urine

Blood that is filtered at the glomerulus travels through the nephron. The nephron is the mainstay of urine formation.

It is composed of:

- The glomerulus
- Proximal convoluted tubule
- Loop of Henle
- Distal convoluted tubule
- Collecting ducts

The glomerulus is where blood is freely filtered. The proximal convoluted tubule is the site where most reabsorption takes place. For example, bicarbonate is freely filtered in the glomerulus but is largely reabsorbed at the proximal convoluted tubule. The loop of Henle is instrumental in concentrating the urine and reabsorbing electrolytes. The distal convoluted tubule leads towards the collecting ducts where water is reabsorbed to produce concentrated urine. The more water the body needs to retain, the more concentrated the urine will be. Acid and base balance is also regulated by the kidneys at the level of the nephron.

Creatinine

Creatinine is the breakdown product of muscle. Creatinine is useful as a measure of renal function because it is freely filtered and not reabsorbed by the nephrons. Therefore, it is fairly accurate measure of clearance or how well the kidneys clear a substance from the serum. Creatinine is measured in the serum and elevations are indicative of renal failure. However, caution must be taken in using creatinine. Foremost, muscle mass is the most important determinant of creatinine levels. A 300-pound body builder will have a higher creatinine than a 75-year-old woman whom has less muscle mass. Furthermore, serum creatinine levels are tougher to interpret in patients with amputations. Therefore, it is imperative to use the Cockcroft-Gault or MDRD equations to accurately assess renal function.

UREA

Urea is the breakdown product of protein metabolism. Proteins are degraded into their component parts by enzymatic reactions and urea is formed as the waste product. Urea is freely filtered at the kidney and is excreted in the urine. When renal failure ensues, urea is not excreted and its levels increase. Urea is measured in the serum as the BUN (blood urea nitrogen). Thus, an indicator for renal failure is an elevated BUN. Moreover, the BUN is used to assess the adequacy of dialysis. Kt/V measures the adequacy of dialysis and the pre- and post-hemodialysis levels of BUN are drawn and factored into the equation.

ALBUMIN

Albumin is the most abundant serum protein in the body. It binds and carries a huge array of compounds including hormones, medications and other proteins. It is also a marker of nutrition. The dialysis patient is at an increased risk of malnutrition. Closely monitoring albumin levels helps the dietitian assess nutritional status. A low albumin level is an indicator of malnutrition and has been associated with increased hospitalization and slower recovery from infections. However, caution must be taken when interpreting albumin levels. A normal albumin does not necessarily indicate proper nutrition. In fact, many dialysis patients have normal albumin levels and remain malnourished.

FLUID SHIFTS IN THE BODY DURING DIALYSIS

Fluid is removed from the body via ultrafiltration. The fluid that is removed comes from the intravascular space. In order to compensate for the intravascular hypovolemia, fluid shifts from the interstitial and intracellular spaces into the blood stream. If the rate of fluid removal (ultrafiltration rate) is too high, fluid will be removed faster than it can be replaced from the interstitium. This will result in hypotension and patients can go into shock. The best method of preventing hypotension is to control the ultrafiltration rate with frequent blood pressure monitoring during dialysis. Furthermore, should hypotension occur, intravenous hypertonic saline could be administered. The hypertonicity will force fluid via osmosis to shift from the interstitial and intracellular spaces into the vasculature. The hypertonic saline would not necessarily correct the hypovolemia directly but will assist in proper fluid shifting.

BIOCOMPATIBILITY

Biocompatibility refers to the body's response when blood interacts with the dialyzer membrane. The dialyzer membrane is a foreign substance. When blood comes into contact with the dialyzer, it will react as if it is being invaded by activating the immune system. The immune system will trigger complement activation (proteins found in the body which activate a cascade of reactions resulting in an immunologic defense). Complement is also a marker for inflammation. The chronic inflammation and complement activation is hazardous to patients and the former is being closely studied today. Cellulose based membranes are less biocompatible than synthetic membranes. The reason synthetic membranes are more biocompatible is that they have fewer antigens on their surface, which the blood recognizes as foreign.

Hemodialysis

HISTORY OF DIALYSIS

The history of "dialysis" began when the London chemist, Thomas Graham, first coined the term in 1861. He gave this name to the process of selective diffusion. In 1913, Abel, Rowntree, and Turner developed a device which utilized collodion tubes through which blood poured while a saline solution washed over the outside of the tubes. This apparatus was implemented successfully in treating animals with uremia. Kolff and Berk later developed an artificial kidney, using the newly developed anticoagulant, heparin and cellophane tubing. In 1948, Skeggs and Leonards invented a parallel plate dialyzer. The first disposable dialyzer, the Travenol twin coil unit, came on the market in 1956. Gambro started production of the disposable parallel plate devices in 1965. Hollow-fiber artificial kidneys were invented at around this same time in the United States.

HEMODIALYSIS

Hemodialysis refers to the process of removing or filtering metabolic wastes out of the blood through a semipermeable membrane. The goal is to supplement the normal functioning of a kidney by managing uremia, fluid overload, and electrolyte imbalance. Molecular size is measured in daltons (DA). Many of the substances that cause uremia have a dalton size of less than 500. These molecules easily diffuse across the cellulose membranes. Particles larger than 500 DA (midsize molecules) diffuse inadequately through these membranes. Large molecules (more than 3000 DA) are not commonly thought to be toxic, except for β_2 microglobulin because of its relationship with bone disease, amyloid, and anemia.

DIALYZERS

There are two main types of dialyzers: parallel plate and hollow fiber. The parallel plate dialyzers work by putting membranes in layers, one on top of the other. The membranes are not flat but are curved with ridges to expand the surface area. The main drawbacks of parallel plate dialyzers are the inability for reuse and compliance (the higher the transmembrane pressure, the higher the volume of blood held). Thus, ultrafiltration cannot be controlled very precisely. The other type of dialyzer is the hollow fiber or HFAK (hollow fiber artificial kidney). This is the most common type of dialyzer used today. It works by having hollow fibers arranged in bundles. They can come in different sizes and thickness and are made of either cellulose or are synthetic. The main advantages of HFAK include being noncompliant and reuse.

HIGH EFFICIENCY AND HIGH FLUX DIALYSIS

High efficiency dialysis refers to cellulosic membranes with increased surface areas. High flux dialysis refers to synthetic membranes with increased surface areas and permeability to larger molecules. The advantage of high flux membranes is their decreased association with cardiovascular events. They also clear β2 microglobulin more efficiently and produce less inflammation by activating complement. They have also been shown to increase patient survival after long-term dialysis treatment (>3.7 years as per the HEMO study). The main problem with high flux dialyzers is that the increased permeability allows for easier access to the patient's bloodstream by gram-negative bacteria.

ARTERIOVENOUS HEMODIALYSIS AND VENOVENOUS HEMODIALYSIS

CAVHD and CVVHD remove solutes and fluid via diffusion. The former uses arterial blood pressure to supply the forces needed to drive blood through the extracorporeal circuit. The latter relies on an external blood pump for flow. A dialysate is used which allows solutes to diffuse down the concentration gradients. Relative to CAVH or CVVH, fluid removal is less efficient. However, solute removal is much better.

ARTERIOVENOUS AND VENOVENOUS TECHNIQUES

Arteriovenous requires both an arterial line and venous line. Arterial blood leaves the body and enters the dialyzer. Blood travels through the dialysis machine under the body's blood pressure. Note that there are no blood pumps providing negative pressure to aid the passage of blood as it travels through the dialyzer. Finally, blood returns to the body via a venous line. Venovenous, on the other hand, only requires a venous line. Blood leaves the body and enters the dialysis machine. However, a blood pump is required to aid the passage of blood. This is because the venous system is a low-pressure system. Blood returns to the body via another lumen into the same large vein.

ADVANTAGES AND DISADVANTAGES

The major advantage to arteriovenous access is its lack of dependence on a blood pump for filtration. This is very important because the patient's blood pressure is supplying the forces of forward flow. A blood pump applies a negative pressure to entice forward flow. The blood pump places the patient at risk for hypotension during the treatment session. The advantage of a venovenous system is that only one vein needs to be punctured for renal replacement and requires less systemic anticoagulation.

The disadvantage of an arteriovenous system includes more anticoagulation, the puncturing of an artery and less reliable blood flow. Again, blood flow is completely reliant on the patient's blood pressure, which can be low in critically ill patients. The disadvantage of a venovenous system is the use of a blood pump (greater chance of hypotension).

CONTINUOUS ARTERIOVENOUS HEMOFILTRATION AND CONTINUOUS VENOVENOUS HEMOFILTRATION

CAVH and CVVH remove solutes and fluid via convection. The former uses arterial blood pressure to supply the forces needed to drive blood through the extracorporeal circuit. The latter relies on an external blood pump for flow. Both operate by removing fluid and solute via convection with replacement fluids to replace excess fluid loss. These techniques are extremely inefficient requiring treatment sessions of up to 24 hours sometimes.

PURIFICATION OF DIALYSIS SOLUTION

Dialysis solution must meet purification standards to avoid patient injury. 120-200 L of dialysis solution comes in direct contact with the patient's blood during dialysis. Small molecular weight contaminants would have access to the bloodstream, possibly causing chemical or microbiologic injury. A purification system must be employed if municipal water is to be used for dialysis. Common contaminants that may be found in water are as follows:

- Aluminum: may cause bone disease, fatal neurologic deterioration, dialysis encephalopathy syndrome, and anemia
- Chloramine: hemolytic anemia
- Fluoride: severe pruritus, nausea, and fatal ventricular fibrillation
- Copper and zinc: hemolytic anemia
- Bacteria and endotoxins: may cause infections and pyrogenic reactions

QUALITY OF DIALYSIS WATER SUPPLY

Meticulous procedures including thorough documentation of the performance of every section of the distribution system must be observed. Standards developed by the AAMI and the European Best Practices Group should be followed in order to maintain optimal patient safety. These include the following:

- Monitor chemical purity of water and dialysis solution.
- Check chloramine levels daily.
- Take chronic toxic component readings in feed water on a regular schedule.
- Measure bacterial growth and endotoxins in water and dialysis fluid using high sensitivity methods.
- Monitor patients for hemolytic, pyrogenic, other reactions, and blood aluminum levels.

A water supply that meets all the standards for the Safe Drinking Water Act and the EPA standards is still not safe for dialysis use. Tap water may be acidic or alkaline, causing problems with the bicarbonate mode of the delivery system maintaining the proper pH. Any contaminants in the water could enter the patient's bloodstream through the dialysis membrane. Substances that may be harmless when water is ingested through the GI system could be toxic if absorbed directly into the blood. Tap water may contain chemicals, organic compounds, nonionic organic compounds, silt, pesticides, herbicides, minerals, microorganisms, trace elements, and endotoxins not found in high-purity water approved for dialysis. The dialyzer membrane cannot distinguish between ions to be absorbed or rejected, making it necessary to eliminate these contaminants prior to their introduction into the dialysis process.

There are many organic and inorganic impurities found in tap water, including chemical solutes, bacteria and their by-products, and particulate matter. Some of the chemicals that can be found in tap water that can be harmful to human beings if found in excess are as follows:

- Chloramines and nitrates: may cause methemoglobinemia in which red blood cells no longer have the ability to carry oxygen
- Copper: may cause hemolysis
- Manganese: toxicity
- Iron: toxicity
- Fluoride: accumulates in bone, aggravates uremic bone disease, toxic to enzyme systems
- Aluminum: accumulates, is related to dialysis-dementia syndrome, anemia and osteodystrophy
- Zinc: GI upset and anemia
- 90Sr: radioactive, poses health danger

ROUTINE TESTS TO ASSURE SAFETY OF WATER TREATMENT SYSTEM

Routine tests that are done on water treatment systems are as follows:

- Conductivity testing is conducted to assure that the feed and product water contains the proper amount of ions. This is done with a Phoenix meter or a Myron-1.
- Bacterial culturing is done to identify any growth in the water or dialysate.
- Resistivity testing is performed to determine the effectiveness of the deionizer.
- Hardness testing determines the amount of calcium and magnesium.
- The total dissolved solids (TDS) measurement verifies the efficiency of the reverse osmosis system by measuring the sum of all the ions in the solution.

TREATMENT OF WATER IN PREPARATION FOR HEMODIALYSIS

Below are ways through which water is treated in preparation for hemodialysis:

- Filtration
- Activated carbon filters (adsorption)
- Water softeners
- Reverse osmosis
- Deionization
- Ultraviolet light exposure

ROLE OF WATER SOFTENERS

The term "water softener" refers to removing calcium and magnesium from the water supply. Thus, "hard water" is water with too much calcium and magnesium. The water softener works by exchanging sodium ions for both calcium and magnesium. The exchange is two sodium for one calcium and two sodium for one magnesium (recall that sodium carries one positive charge and calcium and magnesium are divalent cations). The removal of calcium and magnesium is important in preparing the water prior to further treatment. Other positively charged ions are also removed by the water softener including aluminum.

ROLE OF CARBON TANKS

The carbon tank functions to purify water via activated carbon. The activated carbon helps remove chlorines, chloramines and organic matter via adsorption. There are two carbon tanks at each dialysis facility.

- The first tank is a high flow state that removes most of the chlorine and chloramines.
- The second tank is a low flow state to get any remaining chlorines. The low flow state is more conducive to bacterial growth. Thus, dialysis facilities change the order of tank use daily. Moreover, at the end of each day the tanks must be backwashed so that they can effectively filter the next day. The carbon tanks can be changed entirely by an outside vendor to ensure filter integrity periodically. However, some tanks need not be changed but simply have the carbon filter changed at regular intervals.

ROLE OF DEIONIZATION

Deionization is the process of removing all ions from the water supply. Both cations and anions are removed so that the water used is nonconductive. The process of cation removal involves exchanging hydrogen ions for the cations involved (mostly sodium, potassium, calcium and magnesium). The process of anion removal involves exchanging hydroxide (usually exchanged with chloride, fluoride, sulfate and nitrate). The combination of hydrogen and hydroxide ions combine to form water. However, the major drawback to deionization is that it does not remove endotoxins. Thus, following deionization, a filter or reverse osmosis is needed to remove endotoxins.

ROLE OF REVERSE OSMOSIS

Reverse osmosis is important in freeing water from any leftover contaminants following carbon tanks and water softeners. The water is placed under a high pressure system and is filtered via a semipermeable membrane. The high pressure is needed to ensure that most contaminants, including endotoxins, are picked up while water is forced through the membrane. The water that is emerges is extremely pure and will be held before use for hemodialysis. Reverse osmosis is also referred to as ultrafiltration of the water system. This is not to be confused with the ultrafiltration that occurs during dialysis (removal of excess water from patient's plasma). Rather, this is ultrafiltration at the level of water preparation prior to dialysis treatment.

ROLE OF ULTRAVIOLET LIGHT

Ultraviolet light is used to destroy bacteria contained in water. The light passes through the water and damages the DNA structure of bacteria. It effectively destroys bacteria but does not affect endotoxin. The limitations of ultraviolet light are a need for a low flow state and clarity of water. A low flow state is needed so that the light can effectively penetrate the water. Also, cloudy water distorts ultraviolet light and can lessen its efficacy in eliminating bacteria.

PREPARATION OF DIALYZER FOR USE

Foremost, all dialyzers must be clean of any matter or bacteria when it is received from the manufacturer. The dialyzer should be washed saline solution to clear any leftover particulates. It must also be washed with disinfectant to rid it of any bacteria. Second, it must be free of any air. Air trapped in the dialyzer could easily diffuse into the patient's blood stream and cause an air embolism. Air can also clog the hollow fiber filters and render them ineffective.

PRIMING THE DIALYZER

New and reused dialyzers have to be primed using 500-1000 mL of normal saline solution, depending on the type of unit. All manufacturers have instructions on how to prime their particular dialyzers. Their recommendations should be read and meticulously followed. New units may contain glycerin and particulates that remained from the manufacturing method and will require 1000 mL of saline to ensure that all the contaminants are removed. 500 mL of saline should be sufficient for priming a reused unit with the primer flowing in a counterclockwise pathway to remove any remaining disinfectant.

Removing Air from the Dialyzer

All air needs to be removed from the dialyzer beginning at the bottom. Attach the bloodlines to the dialyzer; turn the dialyzer venous side up and prime with normal saline solution. Next, use the arterial bloodline; infuse the normal saline solution through the dialyzer and out the venous bloodline into a container. As the dialyzer is filled with saline, air will be forced up and out the top. Gently tap the dialyzer and turn it side to side to ensure that all the air is completely out of the header.

Types of Membranes Used in Dialyzers

Don't confuse the type of membranes with type of dialyzers. Parallel and hollow fibers only describe the contour of the membranes and not their composition. Membranes are composed of either cellulose or synthetic. Cellulose is a carbohydrate polymer that is found in plants. It is manufactured to form different thickness and water absorptive qualities and permeabilites. The most common cellulose membrane is cuprophan. The other type of membrane used is synthetically manufactured. The most common types include polyacrylonitrile, polysulfone, polyamide and polymehtyl-methacrylate. They are all easily reused and are noncompliant.

Synthetic Membranes

Synthetic membranes for hemodialysis are thermoplastics, which feature fine, smooth, luminal surfaces sustained by a spongy wall structure. Varieties include polyacrylonitrile (PAN), Polysulfone (P_4S) polyamide, poly-methacrylate (PMMA), and others. Convective transfer accounts for their mass transport.

Advantages of the synthetic membrane are as follows:

- Reusability
- Bioincompatibility

Disadvantages of synthetic membranes include the following:

- Expensive in comparison to cellulose membranes
- High water permeability-ultrafiltration needs to be used
- Absorption of protein to the membrane surface
- Risk of reverse filtration from dialysate to blood

Cellulose Membranes

Cellulose membranes are comprised of a naturally occurring substance. However, that does not necessitate any advantage. Cellulose is cheaper to manufacture and have been in use for a long time. The characteristics of cellulose membranes are better studied than synthetic membranes. However, they cannot be reused and are somewhat bioincompatible (cause an inflammatory response).

Mass Transfer Rate

Mass transfer rate refers to the rate of transfer of solutes across a semipermeable membrane. In dialysis, mass transfer rate applies to the rate of transfer (removal) of toxins and electrolytes, particularly urea and potassium. The mass transfer rate is affected by:

- Temperature
- Surface area of the semipermeable membrane

- Concentration gradient
- Membrane permeability
- Blood
- Dialysate flow rates and flow geometry (usually countercurrent flow)

Mass transfer rates are increased with higher temperatures, greater membrane surface areas and higher concentration gradients.

Countercurrent Flow

Countercurrent flow exists when one fluid is passing in one direction while another fluid is passing in the opposite direction. What separates the two fluids is a semipermeable membrane. In dialysis, blood from the patient flows continuously in one direction while the dialysate solution flows in the opposite direction. The fluids do not intermix and are separated by a semipermeable membrane. The fluids travel in opposite direction to maintain the difference in concentration gradients in the dialyzer. Imagine if both blood and dialysate started at one end of the dialyzer and flowed in the same direction. As they reached the end of the dialyzer the concentration of urea and other electrolytes would equilibrate. However, if the fluids traveled in opposite directions, equilibration would not occur. Urea and other toxins would constantly diffuse from the blood into the dialysate solution down their concentration gradients for the length of the dialyzer.

Physiologic Importance

Countercurrent flow is important in removing toxins and electrolytes from the blood. It allows for a continuous concentration gradient to exist. For example, urea is highly concentrated in blood. As the blood passes through the dialyzer it meets the dialysate solution coming in the opposite direction. Dialysate has a lower urea concentration and thus urea will travel from the blood into the dialysate. The countercurrent flow creates an environment where urea is constantly diffusing down its concentration gradient. The exact same physiology occurs in the kidney where excess toxins and electrolytes are removed in the nephron.

Ultrafiltration

Ultrafiltration refers to hydrostatic pressures forcing plasma volume out of the blood and into the dialysate. Another term for ultrafiltration is transmembrane pressure. Ultrafiltration occurs as follows:

- Blood is delivered to the dialyzer under positive pressure.
- This hydrostatic pressure forces some volume of blood to traverse the semipermeable membrane into the dialysate solution.
- Moreover, dialysate is traveling under negative pressure.
- The negative pressure accentuates the removal of fluid.

It is via ultrafiltration that patients lose the excess water gained between dialysis sessions.

Ultrafiltration Controls

Ultrafiltration controls are used to match the volume of dialysate entering the dialyzer with the volume of dialysate emerging from the dialyzer plus water from the patient. Under normal circumstances, the ultrafiltration will be such that there should be more volume leaving the dialyzer than that entering the dialyzer (recall ultrafiltration is the process of removing excess water from the patient). Parameters are set to the ultrafiltration to govern control of too much or too little volume being removed. There are two types of controls:

- Volumetric
- Flowmetric

VOLUMETRIC AND FLOWMETRIC ULTRAFILTRATION CONTROLS

Volumetric ultrafiltration works by a diaphragm system. As dialysate passes the first diaphragm, an equal volume is delivered to the dialyzer. Then a second diaphragm detects dialysate as it emerges from the dialyzer. As fluid emerges from the dialyzer, an equal volume is delivered to the drain. Flowmetric ultrafiltration works by having detectors of fluid flow in both the inflow and outflow dialysate pathways. Fluid balance is monitored and controlled through the flowmetric monitors.

ISOLATED ULTRAFILTRATION

Isolated ultrafiltration refers to removal of water without solute. The patient is hooked up to the dialysis machine and blood flows through the dialyzer. However, no dialysate is used during the process. Thus, there is little to no solute loss. However, hydrostatic forces are still at play and water is removed from the patient. Ultrafiltration is indicated in patients which are volume overloaded but do not need solute removal i.e. urea, potassium.

REVERSE FILTRATION

Reverse filtration is just the opposite of ultrafiltration. Instead of blood passing under positive pressure and dialysate under negative pressure, the opposite occurs. Now dialysate is under positive pressure while blood is under negative pressure. The danger with reverse filtration is that patients will gain fluid instead of losing it. They will also take on other substances in the dialysate solution such as bicarbonate, potassium and possibly infectious agents (bacteria). Reverse filtration is usually identified via an alarm on the dialysis machine. Dialysis must be immediately stopped if reverse filtration is detected.

RECIRCULATION

Recirculation occurs when blood coming from the dialysis machine is returned to the dialyzer. The arterial systemic circulation should enter the dialyzer and return to the venous side. However, if blood returning from the dialyzer is again circulated back to the dialysis machine, recirculation is taking place. The way to identify recirculation is to obtain an arterial sample from the systemic side and a sample from the arterial line headed towards the dialysis machine. The concentrations of urea should be the same in both samples. If, however, the arterial line has a lower urea concentration than the systemic arterial sample then recirculation is present. Well functioning fistulas should have a recirculation percentage of below 10 percent.

FACTORS THAT AFFECT BLOOD RESISTANCE AS IT FLOWS THROUGH THE DIALYSIS MACHINE

The number one factor affecting blood resistance is the patient's hematocrit. Hematocrit is the main determinant of blood viscosity. The larger the hematocrit, the more viscous and more resistance to blood flow. The other factor in determining blood resistance is the path blood takes as it travels through the dialyzer. The longer the dialyzer the more resistance blood will encounter. The larger the surface area and cross sectional area of the dialyzer, the lower the resistance. These are basic principles of fluid mechanics and a more detailed explanation is provided by Bernoulli's principles. However, for purposes of flow resistance in dialysis the important points to remember are hematocrit and dialyzer length, surface and cross sectional areas.

HEMODIALYSIS AND HEMOFILTRATION

Hemodialysis is the removal of water and solute via diffusion. Blood enters the dialyzer with dialysate flowing in a countercurrent fashion. Solutes diffuse down their concentration gradient from blood to dialysate (removal of urea and potassium). Conversely, calcium and bicarbonate diffuse down their concentration gradient from dialysate to blood. In contrast, hemofiltration does not use diffusion at all. It removes water and solute via convective forces. Dialysate is not used for this technique. Blood enters the dialyzer and small solutes and water are removed under hydrostatic pressure. In order to prevent excess water loss, replacement fluid is needed for hemofiltration. The fluid replacement aids in diluting lost solutes such as urea and potassium and thus their serum levels decrease.

CRRT

Continuous renal replacement therapy (CRRT) is a generic term that applies to various techniques. It operates by removing water and solute via diffusion (dialysis based solute removal) or convection (filtration based solute removal). It is a continuous process and is referred to as a "slow dialysis." There are many techniques in carrying out CRRT and they are essentially categorized based on access. CRRT variations include:

- Slow continuous ultrafiltration (SCUF)
- Continuous arteriovenous hemofiltration (CAVH)
- Continuous arteriovenous hemodialysis (CAVHD)
- Continuous venovenous hemofiltration (CVVH)
- Continuous venovenous hemodialysis (CVVHD)

For CAVH and CAVHD, arterial access is required. For all others there is no need for arterial access as double lumen catheters are placed in large veins. However, CVVH and CVVHD require a blood pump during the procedure.

BLOOD PUMP READINGS

Blood pumps that have rate indicators display the flow determined by the speed of rotation. The variables that could affect the accuracy of the blood pump's readings are as follows:

- Internal diameter of tubing: must match that which was used for calibrating the pump
- Pressure conditions in blood circuit
- Lack of linearity across indicator scale
- Type of tubing used

The calibration process should be done on a regular basis, under standard conditions, with the exact brand and lot of tubing that is being used clinically. The water used should be at 37° C, pumped from the source through partially clamped tubing to approximate the negative pressure between the needle and the dialysis pump. A graduated cylinder should be used for holding the outflow solution, and it should be collected over a 3 to 5-minute period. The resulting volume in millimeters divided by the time in minutes gives the flow rate.

ULTRASONIC AIR/FOAM DETECTOR

The ultrasonic air/foam detector is a commonly used type of apparatus for detection the presence of air. It uses ultrasonic beams to find air, foam, or microbubbles in the blood. Since sound traverses liquid more rapidly than air, even minute levels of air will disrupt the sonic beam and trigger the alarm. The alarm system of most ultrasonic detectors may be disarmed while priming and rinsing the dialysis delivery system. When the alarm system is inactive, a constant, low-level alarm should be sounding, to indicate the disarmed state. Dialysis should never be performed on a patient when the air/foam detector is not activated.

Blood Leak Monitors

Blood leaks occur when blood traverses the semipermeable membrane and flows with the dialysate. As dialysate leaves the dialyzer it passes over a light sensor. If the light is obstructed from reaching its sensor via a change in fluid composition (i.e. blood), then an alarm sounds. Locating where the blood leak occurs is crucial and dialysis is temporarily halted. Obviously, blood leaking into the system will have serious effects on the patient including hypotension, electrolyte imbalance and possibly death.

Dialyzer Reuse

Dialyzer reuse is the process of sterilizing the dialyzer after it is used. Dialyzer reuse is authorized for the same patient only. For infection control purposes, dialyzers are not allowed to be cleaned and reused on different patients. The main advantage of reuse is lower costs and fewer first pass side effects (each dialyzer is different and each time one is introduced, patients may experience side effects).

The disadvantages of reuse include:

- Expensive sterilizing techniques
- Hazardous sterilizing materials and chemicals
- Quality control to ensure proper dialyzer storage and to ensure it is reused in the same patient only

The following are the four main criteria used to determine dialyzer reusability:

- Total cell volume – most common method to determine dialyzer reusability. The dialyzer is initially filled with water and then emptied (before being used on a patient). Then after hemodialysis the dialyzer is again filled with water and emptied. The emptied water must measure at least 80% of the initial water volume. If it is less than eighty percent, the dialyzer is not fit for reuse.
- Pressure testing – also referred to as leak testing. This test ensures there is no blood leak during dialysis. Pressure is applied to the dialyzer. If the pressure falls, then there is a leak and the dialyzer is not fit for use.
- Ultrafiltration coefficient – used as an indirect measure of how well dialyzers clear substances. This is not to be confused with clearance but rather a test of the membrane's permeability.
- Visual inspection – Examining the dialyzer for large blood streaks indicates clotted membranes and not fit for use.

The process in cleaning a dialyzer prior to reuse is described below:

- The dialyzer is first flushed with saline to remove left over blood products.
- Then a cleanser is added to clear all contaminants including bacteria.
- After cleaning and disinfecting, the dialyzer is tested for integrity of use. The membrane must still be intact and capable of removing waste.
- Finally, a disinfectant is used as a final step to clear all contaminants and waste.

SDS

The method used to deliver solutions used to produce dialysate to the machine is called the SDS, or solution delivery system. The overhead holding tank is referred to as the "head" tank. Bicarbonate from a mixing tank and acid from a storage tank are transferred to the head tank. These solutions are gravity fed to a solution distribution system (SDS) and then routed to the treatment area where it enters a series of pipes attached to the dialysis machines. Some supply only one patient while other solution delivery systems supply several dialyzers at the same time.

DIALYSATE

Dialysate is a solution, prepared as a chemical composition, to be as similar to normal plasma as possible. It carries away waste materials and excess fluid extracted from the blood by the dialysis process. Dialysate prevents the depletion of essential electrolytes and prevents the removal of excess water. The five chemicals that are most frequently used to make dialysate are as follows:

- Sodium chloride
- Sodium bicarbonate or sodium acetate
- Calcium chloride
- Potassium chloride
- Magnesium chloride

In some cases, glucose is also added to the formulation.

PRIMARY AND SECONDARY TESTS TO ASSURE THE COMPOSITION OF DIALYSATE

The primary test calculates the concentration of a solute by the laboratory method called reliability. Two such tests are flame photometry for testing sodium content and titration to find chloride. This type of analysis is important to assure the proper ratio of acid to bicarbonate and to determine the ratio of concentrate to water. The secondary test uses overall conductivity. Most suppliers of concentrate indicate on the label the proper level of conductivity that should be seen when the solution is properly mixed. Another secondary test measures total osmolality by freezing-point depression or vapor pressure to determine the total amount of solute in the dialysate.

PROPORTIONING SYSTEMS

Proportioning systems, most of which use microprocessor circuitry to control the pace of the proportioning pumps and the volume of concentrates added, ensure that the dialysis fluid is properly mixed. The advantages of the proportioning systems are as follows:

- These systems mix fixed volumes of dialysate concentrates with fixed volumes of heated purified water or use conductivity-based servo control systems to mix the concentrates and water.
- Ionic composition of the final dialysate is checked by conductivity.
- If the conductivity is outside the proper range, alarms sound and dialysis stops.

The main disadvantages of proportioning systems are as follows:

- Expense of the units
- Preprogrammed functions may be difficult to change
- Sensors and monitoring devices must reliable and redundant
- Difficult to troubleshoot
- May need factory representative for repairs

DEAERATION DEVICES

Deaeration devices are used on dialysate solution. Water from a public water source is below room temperature and needs to be heated before being delivered to the dialyzer, usually at 35°-38° C. Microbubbles and dissolved air are found in water. As the temperature increases, the air trapped in the water is released as expanding microbubbles. These microbubbles negatively affect conductivity sensors, temperature and flowmeters. These bubbles also diminish the contact of the dialysate and membrane in hollow-fiber dialyzers. To release the dissolved air from the solution, deaeration devices use a combination of heat and negative pressure. These air bubbles are trapped by a coalescing filter then vented to the outside.

"A" AND "B" CONCENTRATE

The "A" concentrate contains a high level of sodium, along with calcium, magnesium, potassium, chloride, and a minimal amount of acetic acid. The "B" (bicarbonate) concentrate is made of the sodium bicarbonate. In some systems, a portion of the sodium chloride is mixed into this solution to increase its overall conductivity, producing a concentrate that is simple to monitor. In the proportioning system, the "B" concentrate is frequently diluted with water, while the "A" concentrate is then mixed in and the resulting fluid flows into the dialyzer. In the closed system, CO_2 is unable to be released as bubbles; therefore, the reaction between the sodium bicarbonate and the acetic acid cannot come to fruition, and the hydrogen ion content keeps the calcium in solution.

SVS

The sodium variation system (SVS), also known as sodium modeling, is a device that may be instituted to decrease some of the complications of hemodialysis treatment, specifically, cramping and hypotension. In rapid dialysis, the fluid is depleted from the intravascular space, and the replenishing of this fluid may not happen quickly enough to prevent hypotension. When the blood pressure falls, cramping of the arms and legs occurs due to their decreased vascular volume. Hypoalbuminemia and right-sided heart failure may also play a part in the delayed refilling of this fluid. The SVS uses a computer model of sodium and water movement between compartments during the hemodialysis procedure. The sodium content varies during the treatment by either adding a special NaCl concentrate or by varying the proportion of the usual concentrate.

SORBENT REGENERATIVE SYSTEM

The sorbent regenerative system uses a cartridge of absorbent materials through which dialysate is recirculated and chemically regenerated. This process removes metabolic wastes from the dialysate and the pH and electrolyte content are restored. This system performs these actions:

- Converts urea to ammonium carbonate
- Absorbs creatinine and other nonionized solutes
- Ion exchange resins (sodium zirconium phosphate and zirconium oxide)

The contents of the four chambers of the sorbent regenerative cartridge are as follows:

- Activated carbon
- Hydrated zirconium oxide
- Zirconium phosphate
- Urease

ADVANTAGES AND DISADVANTAGES

The advantages of the sorbent system are as follows:

- Portability
- No need for special water supply
- No need for special drainage connections
- Adaptable to various electrical systems

The disadvantages of the sorbent system are as follows:

- Expensive cartridge
- Limit on capacity to eliminate urea
- Limit on capacity to absorb ammonia
- Ammonia may build-up in the system and in the patient
- Large patients with high urea levels may need additional cartridge

ADDITIONAL EQUIPMENT NEEDED DURING DIALYSIS

The additional equipment needed for dialysis includes the following:

- Blood pump with blood flow rate
- Heparin infusion pump
- Air/foam detector
- Inflow and outflow pressure sensors

BICARBONATE

Bicarbonate dialysate is the standard of practice in most dialysis facilities. The diffusion of bicarbonate acts as a buffer to the hydrogen ions during hemodialysis and aids in the acid-base balance. Since one of the goals of hemodialysis is to correct acidosis associated with renal failure, sodium bicarbonate concentrate is added to the dialysate as one of the three streams of fluid used. The concentrate comes packaged in two sections. One is "acid concentrate" and the other is "bicarbonate concentrate".

The three streams of fluid are as follows:

- Water, 34 parts
- Acid concentrate, 1 part
- Bicarbonate concentrate, 1.8 parts

Different types of equipment use concentrates of varying compositions. Mismatched concentrate may lead to a fatal error.

DIALYSATE SOLUTION FUNCTION

Dialysate solution functions to remove urea, certain electrolytes and other wastes from the blood. It must also ensure to not remove other electrolytes or excess water. It accomplishes this by being near identical to serum in its electrolyte concentrations. Dialysate is mostly composed of the following: sodium chloride, sodium bicarbonate or sodium acetate, calcium chloride, potassium chloride and magnesium chloride. Most concentrations of these solutions are standard with the exception of potassium chloride. The potassium concentration is dictated with the dialysis orders based on serum potassium levels. Higher serum potassium will necessitate greater removal and thus a lower potassium dialysate concentration.

MONITORING DIALYSATE CONCENTRATION

Dialysate concentration is monitored by the conductivity monitor. The conductivity monitor senses total electrolyte or ion flow in the dialysate solution. The conductivity monitor cannot sense individual electrolyte concentrations (e.g. Na concentration of dialysate). However, it can detect total electrolyte flow. Conductivity monitors essentially function just like batteries with monitoring occurring as electrolytes flow past them. Just like batteries, over time they run out and must be replaced. The purpose of conductivity is to ensure that electrical current is not circulating through the dialysis apparatus and transferred to the patient.

Controlling Dialysate Temperature

Foremost, dialysate temperature should be kept at near normal body temperature. A cold dialysate can cause hypothermia for the patient. Conversely, a hot dialysate can cause hypotension and hemolysis. During dialysis water is removed causing a hypovolemia. The body's natural response is to vasoconstrict to maintain blood pressure. If the dialysate is too warm, the body's ability to vasoconstrict is limited and hypotension ensues. Also, hot dialysate can lead to hemolysis, which can persist for hours. The temperature of the dialysate is set and monitored by the machine and should be kept at around 36 degrees Celsius.

LAL Test

LAL is short for limulus amebocyte lysate. It is a test of the water dialysate to check for endotoxins. Endotoxins are found with gram-negative bacteria. Because the water system used for dialysate is not sterile, gram-negative bacteria can contaminate the water. Dialysate with gram-negative bacteria can lead to severe complications including sepsis and patient death. The LAL test is performed daily to ensure the water system is negative for bacteria.

Factors That Affect Removal of Toxins

During dialysis, there are several factors that affect the successful removal of toxins. Six of the factors that affect the successful removal of toxins are as follows:

- Temperature of the dialysate: higher temperature = more solutes removed
- Flow rate: faster dialysate flow rate = greater removal of solutes
- Molecular weight of solutes: lower molecular weight = more solute removal
- Concentration gradient: higher concentration = higher diffusion
- Membrane permeability: more permeable membrane = greater removal of solutes
- Blood flow rate: greater blood flow = greater removal of solutes

The term semipermeable membrane refers to a membrane that allows certain substances to filter through while separating out others. Large molecules are retained in the membrane while smaller molecules easily traverse.

Viscosity of the Blood

Hematocrit levels affect the viscosity (thickness and stickiness) of the blood. The greater the number of RBC's in the blood, the higher the hematocrit level. Centipoise is the term used to measure the viscosity of a liquid. Blood with a 30% hematocrit level is around 2.5 centipoise, or about 2.5 times as viscous as water.

Geometry Aspects of Blood Pathway

The "geometric" properties of the blood pathway are the physical properties, such as length, width, surfaces, cross-sections, etc. Geometric aspects include the following:

- The length of the pathway is important, short pathways (15-50 cm) as in the hollow-fiber dialyzers offer low resistance.
- The number of pathways affect the resistance, the higher the number, the lower the resistance, e.g. hollow-fiber dialyzers with thousands of pathways have very low resistance.

The cross-sectional area of a pathway plays a significant role; the larger the cross-sectional pathway, the lower the amount of resistance. In hollow-fiber dialyzers, the internal radius is the control factor.

INITIATING HEMODIALYSIS IN PATIENTS WITHOUT CHRONIC KIDNEY DISEASE STAGE V

The following are reasons for initiating hemodialysis in patients who do not have Chronic Kidney Disease Stage V:

- Volume overload
- Metabolic acidosis
- Uremic Encephalopathy
- Refractory Hypertension
- Hyperkalemia
- Hyper or Hypocalcemia
- Pericarditis
- Ingestion of dialyzable products

Complications

The most common complications that occur during dialysis treatment are as follows:

- Hypotension
- Cramping
- Nausea and vomiting
- Headache
- Chest pain
- Back pain
- Itching
- Fever and chills

DRY WEIGHT

The term "dry weight" refers to the postdialysis weight at which the patient has had all of his or her excess body fluid removed. If the measurement of dry weight is set too high, the patient will continue to be in a fluid-overloaded state after the dialysis treatment. This could result in edema or pulmonary congestion. If the number is too low, the patient may experience hypotension in the latter part of the dialysis treatment and complain of cramping, dizziness, and malaise after the treatment is complete.

ACUTE RENAL FAILURE IN PEDIATRIC PATIENTS

Special considerations must be given to children undergoing hemodialysis. The pediatric dialysis nurse needs to have a thorough understanding of pediatric nursing plus childhood growth and development. In addition, a comprehensive knowledge of the causes of both acute renal failure and chronic renal failure is imperative. Some of the most common causes for acute renal failure in the pediatric patient include the following:

- Septic shock - resulting in hypoperfusion of the kidneys
- Hypotension - causing hypoperfusion of the kidneys
- Severe dehydration - from gastroenteritis or acute blood loss from surgery or an accident, also results in hypoperfusion
- Acute tubular necrosis - from nephrotoxic drugs such as aminoglycoside, antibiotics, and amphotericin B
- Hemolytic uremic syndrome - most common cause of acute renal failure in children in North America

Although acute poststreptococcal glomerulonephritis is frequently seen in the pediatric population, it rarely results in the need for dialysis.

Comorbid Conditions That Can Complicate ESRD Treatment in Patients

Comorbid conditions in the elderly dialysis patients that complicate treatment for ESRD include the following:

- Cardiovascular disease
- Diabetes
- Reduced protein intake and delayed protein synthesis
- Osteoporosis
- Pulmonary disease
- Impaired vision
- Poor mobility
- Cognition difficulties
- Lack of coordination
- Socioeconomic and psychosocial issues/although not physical, complicate treatment

Advantages of in-Center Treatment for Older Patients

Advantages of in-center hemodialysis for the elderly patient are numerous and consist of the following:

- Social interaction with dialysis personnel
- Frequent observation by medical personnel to assess patient
- Early recognition and intervention for complications
- In-center treatment is safe and comfortable

Predialysis Assessment of Risk Factors

The condition of the patient at the time dialysis is initiated plays a crucial role in survival rate. Several risk factors need to be assessed before the patient begins dialysis. These include the control of the following:

- Blood pressure
- Anemia
- Calcium/phosphorus intake
- Nutrition during the predialysis period

Comprehensive Predialysis Program

The areas that should be addressed in a comprehensive, multidisciplinary predialysis program include the following:

- Patient and family education
- Choice of suitable modality
- Access of dialysis
- Advantages of fewer urgent dialyses
- Fewer hospital stays in 1st month after beginning dialysis
- Significant cost savings after beginning dialysis

Membrane Biocompatibility

Inflammatory responses occur when blood contacts a foreign surface. If the reaction is severe with a high level of inflammation, the membrane is bioincompatible. When the reaction is mild, the membrane is biocompatible. The complement system consists of a series of plasma proteins that react consecutively to start a series of biological occurrences. The immune system reacts to the foreign substance, the membrane, as it would to a bacterial challenge. Markers are used to evaluate the level of reaction, or the complement activation. These are C3a, C5a, which are used to describe complement activation, and C5b through C9 in the patient's blood.

LONG-TERM USE OF BIOINCOMPATIBLE AND BIOCOMPATIBLE MEMBRANES FOR HEMODIALYSIS

The possible negative effects of long-term usage of bioincompatible membranes are increased incidence of the following:

- Infection
- Malignancy
- Damaged nutritional state
- β_2 Amyloid disease

Probable reasons for the higher incidences of these negative outcomes include the following:

- Cellulose membranes are incapable of removing large β_2-Microglobulin molecules
- Due to cellulose membranes causing increased complement generation, some products of this may cause the release of β_2 from monocytes

Clinical manifestations that may result are as follows:

- Bone lesions
- Arthropathies
- Pathological fractures
- Soft tissue edema
- Carpal tunnel syndrome

REACTION OF THE BODY TO CELLULOSE MEMBRANES

The similarity of the cellulose surface to the cell wall of bacteria, with both being composed of polysaccharide structures, causes the body to react as if it were being attacked by bacteria. The main sources of the extreme complement activation are the free hydroxyl groups on the membrane surface. In order to diminish this reaction, chemical alterations are employed to buffer these free hydroxyl groups, producing "modified cellulosic membranes," such as cellulose acetate and Hemophan. Both modified membranes reduce the reaction, but neither is as effective as a synthetic membrane in diminishing the complement production.

Patients with some residual renal function may be negatively affected by the use of cellulose membranes. The theory postulates that the use of hemodialysis membranes that are more compatible and do not trigger complement activation leads to better recovery and survival rates. The lower the incidence of complement activation, the fewer white cells are produced and the less inflammation results. In one study, patients who were on hemodialysis with cellulose acetate membranes seemed to lose their residual renal function at a faster rate than patients who were dialyzed with a polysulfone membrane.

The practice of dialyzer reuse by the same patient after the cleaning and sterilizing of the equipment has been followed for many years. When proper techniques are used, this is a safe and cost-effective method.

Problems Associated with Internal AV Fistulas

The most common problems associated with internal AV fistulas are as follows:

- The length of time needed for veins to be sufficiently enlarged may be an issue as this process usually takes about 6 weeks.
- Obtaining the desired blood flow may be difficult; dilation may occur in the veins on the back of the hand instead of the forearm in side-to-side anastomoses. This may require surgical correction.
- Vessel spasm causes decreased arterial flow.
- Venous stenosis or needle position may cause return-flow resistance.
- Accidental injury to the vessel during venipuncture may result in hematoma and the inability to use this site for days.
- In "radial artery steal" syndrome the radial artery has a lower arterial pressure, and the pressure gradient causes the ulnar artery blood to flow into the fistula instead of the hand and fingers, which become painful and cold. This may be surgically corrected.
- Infections are common.
- Thrombosis is the most common complication.
- Aneurysms may occur.

Black Blood Syndrome

A fistula with low blood flow rate may lead to recirculation. This low blood flow rate is often the result of stenosis at one of the ends of the fistula and is associated with an increase in venous pressure. Recirculation may lead to "black blood syndrome" in which the blood's acidity level increases, causing the red blood cells to lose their ability to transport oxygen. When the pH of the blood is below 7, it appears very dark in color. To test for this, 3 blood samples are taken, one from a peripheral (P) source, one from the inflow line just before it enters the dialyzer (arterial, A), and one from the outflow line just after it leaves the dialyzer (venous, V). Recirculation should remain at under 10%; if more than 15%, it is excessive and should be investigated and corrected.

Negative Outcomes of Using a Catheter for Dialysis

Venous catheters and traditional hemodialysis access sites may be used for dialysis. Patients using venous catheters may experience the following:

- A higher likelihood of infection
- Increased levels of inflammatory markers, such as C-reactive protein
- A higher mortality rate, which could be due to different patient populations, risks from receiving catheters, or some property of catheter use
- Inadequate blood flow through venous catheters
- Lower than average urea reduction rate (URR) in larger patients
- Fractional urea clearance (Kt/V) in large patients
- Lower survival rate (for catheters around 60% at 6 months and 40% at one year, if revisions are done)

Preventing Hypotension

Hypotension is the most common complication seen during dialysis. Preventative measures that can be used to help avoid the complication of hypotension during dialysis are as follows:

- The ultrafiltration controller closely controls the fluid removal rate. If it is unavailable, use a membrane with low permeability to water so that transmembrane pressure fluctuations will remain small.

- Avoid interdialytic weight gain and instruct the patient to limit salt intake.
- Increase treatment time.
- Use care in determining "dry weight."
- Use correct dialysis solution sodium level.
- Maintain proper dialysate temperature.
- Avoid intradialytic food ingestion.
- Perform a predialysis test for a hemoglobin level of more than 11 g/dL (110 g/L).
- Maintain therapeutic dialysate calcium concentration (especially in cardiac patients).
- Administer antihypertensive medications after dialysis treatment, not before.

Preventing Hypotensive Episodes and Cramping

Medications and some techniques that may be effective in the prevention of hypotensive episodes and cramping during dialysis are as follows:

- Quinine sulfate may be used to prevent cramping.
- Carnitine, oxazepam, or prazosin may reduce cramping during dialysis, although prazosin may cause hypotension.
- Stretching exercises may be beneficial in preventing cramping in certain muscles.
- Sequential compression devices may help reduce leg cramping.

The elements in the blood that need to be at appropriate levels prior to dialysis treatment are as follows:

- Magnesium
- Calcium
- Potassium

Raising the dialysis sodium level just below the level that would cause postdialysis thirst would also help with prevention of cramping.

Severe Hypotension

Steps that should be taken in cases of severe hypotension that occurs during dialysis treatment are as follows:

- Place the patient in the Trendelenburg position (feet up, head down).
- Administer a bolus of 0.9% saline, 100mL or more, through the bloodline (if respiratory status tolerates).
- Reduce the ultrafiltration rate to near zero.

Muscle Cramps During Dialysis

Dialysis patients frequently experience muscle cramps during the first months of treatment. Factors that may contribute to muscle cramps are as follows:

- Hypotension
- Hypovolemia
- High ultrafiltration rate
- Low sodium dialysis solution
- Hypomagnesemia
- Hypocalcemia
- Hypokalemia

REVERSE FILTRATION

Reverse filtration occurs when the dialysate solution moves into the blood. This creates an unsafe condition since the water used for dialysate solution is not sterile. Bicarbonate concentrate, which may be added, promotes the growth of bacteria. Toxins and breakdown products could transfer through the membrane and into the patient's bloodstream. As a result, infections and other unfavorable reactions may develop. A molecular filter (ultrafilter) device can be used to eradicate unwanted molecular particles while allowing dissolved solutes to pass through. This filter would remove bacteria and pyrogens from the solution.

There is a possibility of reverse filtration occurring at the distal end of the dialyzer during high-flux dialysis. If reverse filtration happens during high-flux dialysis, the limulus amebocyte lysate (LAL) test is performed to determine what, if any, endotoxins are present. This test uses endotoxin units (EU) or nanograms per mL (1ng/mL=5 EU/mL). No more than 200 colony forming units (CFU) per mL of water, or 2 EU by LAL, may be present in order to meet AAMI standards.

Counter measures to ensure the safety of high-flux dialysis include the following:

- Installation of a molecular filter or ultrafilter in the dialysate line just ahead of the dialyzer may be used to filter out endotoxins
- Use of high-purity water from enhanced membrane reverse osmosis systems

ULTRAFILTRATION PROFILING

The process of ultrafiltration may result in a sudden reduction of fluid in the vascular compartment. Ultrafiltration profiling refers to the ability of certain dialysis machines to fluctuate the volume of fluid removal during the treatment. The machine automatically divides the total volume to be removed (determined by the nurse) by the length of the treatment. When the ultrafiltration rate is excessive, hypovolemia and hypotension may result. In order to avoid this outcome, the use of hypertonic saline, which enhances the osmolality in the extravascular and vascular spaces, is recommended. This hypertonic solution draws fluid form the vast intracellular reservoir, avoiding the hypovolemia that leads to hypotension.

CARPAL TUNNEL SYNDROME

Carpal tunnel syndrome (CTS), median neuropathy, is a compression of the median nerve at the wrist by the thickened sheath of the carpal tunnel. The cause of this thickening, in dialysis patients, is the amyloid deposition in the sheath. Carpal tunnel syndrome leads to numbness and muscle weakness in the hand, especially the thumb, index, and middle fingers. The hallmark of this syndrome is pain or numbness and tingling in these regions at night. Treatment consists of nonsteroidal anti-inflammatory drugs (NSAIDS) and ultrasound therapy. Kidney transplantation frequently leads to a prompt cessation of symptoms.

CLINICAL MANIFESTATIONS OF INTRADIALYTIC COMPLEMENT ACTIVATION

The clinical manifestations of intradialytic complement activation are as follows:

- Leukopenia, a sharp drop in white cells, that corrects itself after 15 minutes and is nearly normal at the end of 4 hours, is important in patients with compromised cardiac or pulmonary function.
- C5a, the end product of the complement cascade, activates the white cells to be released and to clump, usually in the lungs.
- This reaction reduces the patient's ability to exchange O_2 and CO_2 and may result in hypoxemia.
- Symptoms of chest pain, back pain, coagulation abnormalities, and anaphylaxis may be seen.
- This reaction peaks at 15 minutes but may last up to 90 minutes.

BICARBONATE DIALYSATE

POTENTIAL PROBLEMS

Bicarbonate dialysate is an unstable solution. It requires the addition of a stabilizer, such as a polymer or dry $NaHCO_4$ powder. It is also vulnerable to bacterial contamination and once mixed the solution must be used within 24 hours. Proper sanitation of all containers and mixing apparatus is imperative to avoid contamination of the solution.

WATER USED FOR PREPARATION

The water used for preparation of the B (bicarbonate) dialysate has to meet Advancement of Medical Instrumentation (AAMI) standards regarding the chemical make-up and pyrogen and bacterial content in order to be considered "dialysis-quality water". The microbial count has to register as less than 200 CFU/mL, and the endotoxin concentration has to be less than 2EU/mL.

INFUSION OF AIR DURING DIALYSIS

When a patient receives an infusion of air during dialysis, the following steps must be taken immediately:

- Clamp the bloodlines.
- Discontinue dialysis.
- Position the patient on the left side in the Trendelenburg position (head down, feet up); this decreases air movement to the brain, traps air in the right atrium above the tricuspid valve, and diminishes foaming in right ventricle.
- Maintain the airway and administer oxygen, if necessary.
- Keep the patient still and in this position for several hours for reabsorption of nitrogen and other gases.
- Obtain a chest x-ray to assess the presence of air in the heart.

CAUSES OF CHEST PAIN

Chest pain should always be treated as cardiac in origin until proven otherwise. Dialysis patients are at increased risk for myocardial infarctions and other coronary related events. A complete history and physical must be performed with particular attention to cardiac risk factors: hypertension, diabetes mellitus, hyperlipidemia, age, history of smoking, history of stroke or heart attack, peripheral vascular disease. An electrocardiogram should be urgently done with cardiac enzymes drawn. Oxygen supplementation, morphine, nitrates, aspirin and beta blockers should also be administered. Other causes of chest pain include hemolysis, air embolism, pulmonary embolism, and hypotension.

CAUSES OF HEADACHE, NAUSEA AND VOMITING

Longer dialysis sessions and excess urea removal are frequently a root cause for headaches, nausea and vomiting. A more ominous presentation of a headache with nausea and vomiting is a myocardial infarction or early stroke. Dialysis patients are at increased risk for coronary events and this presentation may be the earliest and only signs of an impending event. Proper risk stratification with attention given to a history of hypertension, diabetes, coronary artery disease, and stroke should prompt early intervention. The dialysis disequilibrium syndrome is a rare cause of headaches. Urea removal may cause a reverse osmosis into the brain, which will cause cerebral swelling presenting as headaches and nausea. Less aggressive dialysis sessions should be curative. Other causes of headache, nausea and vomiting include caffeine withdrawal, migraine or tension headaches, metabolite disturbances (hypoglycemia, hypo and hypernatremia), medications and withdrawal from medicines.

CAUSES OF ITCHING

Itching is a very common complaint of dialysis patients. There are two main reasons:

- The first is an unknown complication of chronic dialysis patients.
- The second could be an indication of inadequate dialysis and thus a sign of uremia.

Frequent measuring of Kt/V would indicate the adequacy of treatments. Other causes of itching include allergies to latex and medications.

CAUSES OF BACK PAIN

Back pain is not very specific to any particular complication but is a common complaint. Hemolysis can present as back pain as well as conditions related to the musculoskeletal system. It is also not uncommon for back pain to present as a coronary event or indigestion.

CAUSES OF HEMOLYSIS

Hemolysis frequently presents as chest pressure, back pain and headaches. If hemolysis is suspected, urgent intervention is needed to prevent hyperkalemia. Dialysis should be immediately stopped and the root cause found. Hemolysis usually occurs with problems with the dialysis solutions. This includes:

- Overheating
- Hypotonicity
- Contamination by formaldehyde, bleach, chloramines, nitrates, and copper

The water system must be rigorously reviewed and the solutions sent for analysis of tonicity. Other causes of hemolysis include red blood cell trauma. All lines must be examined for kinks and improper clamping.

CAUSES OF FEVERS AND CHILLS

Fevers and chills are frequently found in dialysis patients. The most common cause is an infection with the most common origin being the access site. Permcaths, fistulas and AV grafts are excellent sources of staphylococcus and streptococcus introductions into the blood stream. A patient with fevers, chills, hypotension or simply "toxic looking" needs two sets of blood cultures and urgent broad-spectrum antibiotics with hospitalization. Other sources of infections include viral upper respiratory infections, pneumonia, endocarditis and cellulitis. Fevers may also stem from adverse reactions to medications, allergic reactions and other inflammatory states (e.g. coronary events, gout).

CAUSES OF ARRHYTHMIA

Arrhythmias are common in dialysis patients with the most common being ventricular arrhythmias. Treatment with varying concentrations of potassium solutions may be precipitate ventricular arrhythmias. Risk factors for arrhythmias include coronary artery disease and left ventricular cardiomyopathy. Arrhythmias are also precipitated by rapid changes in electrolyte balances during dialysis particularly potassium, calcium and magnesium. Frequent monitoring of pulse and rhythm will help the clinician identify arrhythmias early. The most dangerous rhythm is a sustained wide complex tachycardia. This is usually a ventricular tachycardia but other rhythms are possible. Wide complex tachycardia needs to be treated according to current ACLS guidelines. Supraventricular tachycardias are also common and treatment with adenosine or nodal blocking agents may be appropriate. Electroconversion is reserved for those patients with hypotension.

Disequilibrium Syndrome

Disequilibrium syndrome occurs when urea is removed quickly from the patient. Urea is a major osmole in the body and its removal will cause a fluid shift from the hypoosmolar blood to the hyperosmolar cells. This is particularly concerning in brain cells and fluid shifts will cause cerebral edema and possibly brain damage. Symptoms include tremors, disorientation and convulsions. Treatment of disequilibrium includes halting dialysis and administering hypertonic saline, glucose and mannitol.

Dialyzer Reaction

Dialyzer reaction occurs when the patient is first exposed to dialysis. They develop an allergic reaction and there are two forms: type A and type B.

- Type A is more severe and consists of an anaphylactoid reaction, which includes dyspnea, chest and back pain, respiratory rate increase, hypotension and possibly death. Type A reactions are usually due to exposure to ethylene oxide, a substance used in disinfecting dialyzers.
- Type B reactions are less similar but can present similarly. Treatment includes halting dialysis and administration of antihistamines.

Formaldehyde Reaction

The formaldehyde reaction occurs when the patient's blood is exposed to formaldehyde. Formaldehyde is commonly used to disinfect dialyzers. When dialyzers are not properly rinsed residual formaldehyde can remain. Symptoms to formaldehyde exposure include: bitter taste, perioral numbness, chest and back pain and shortness of breath. Dialysis should be stopped.

B2 Microglobulin Amyloidosis in Patients on Dialysis

β2 microglobulin amyloidosis is a condition that is unique to patients on long-term hemodialysis and occurs rarely in patients on peritoneal dialysis. β2 microglobulin is a polypeptide that accumulates and deposits in patient's joints and tissues. Patients present with joint pain and immobility, carpal tunnel syndrome, skeletal spine immobility and gastrointestinal and heart defects. The exact etiology of the amyloidosis is unclear. The only known treatment is transplant.

Referral for Evaluation When an Access Clot Is Suspected

Foremost, any abnormal finding with measurement techniques such as ultrasound or MRA should not prompt immediate evaluation. It is better to obtain serial measurements and conduct a trend analysis (with each measurement there is less flow suggesting stenosis). For AV grafts an access flow rate of less than 600 mL/min should prompt a referral. For fistulae the access flow rate should be 400- 500 mL/min. Other measurements include a venous segment static pressure ratio of greater than 0.5 in both grafts and fistulae and an arterial segment static pressure ratio greater than 0.75 in grafts. Access recirculation or inadequate dialysis (as defined by a Kt/V or Urea reduction ratio) should also lead to access evaluation. Finally, and most importantly, any indication of limb ischemia at the access site requires emergent evaluation by a vascular surgeon.

Dialysis Catheter Dysfunction

Dialysis catheters are said to be dysfunctional or under functioning when the blood flow rate is less than 300 mL/min. Dysfunctional catheters should be treated via the following methods:

- Repositioning: Sometimes catheters can get stuck or are lodged in next to the venous wall. This will obstruct flow and repositioning the catheter will free it from adhering to the wall. Thrombolytics are indicated when there is a suspected clot in the catheter. Usually heparin is administered with each dialysis session to prevent clot formation but it is not absolute. Small thrombolytic doses can aid in breaking up a clot.
- Catheter Exchange: If the aforementioned measures fail, a catheter exchange may be needed.

Treatment for Infections of AV Grafts and Fistulae

AV graft and fistulae infections should be treated immediately. Dialysis through infected access sites is contraindicated. The antibiotic of choice should cover both gram negative and gram-positive bacteria. Prior to antibiotics, blood cultures should be drawn. Subsequent antibiotics should be based on culture and sensitivity results. Antibiotics have to be administered intravenously to be efficacious. If the infection does not resolve, incision and drainage or complete AV graft or fistula removal may be necessary.

Treatment for Infected Dialysis Catheters

Dialysis catheter infections are suggested when the patient presents with fever, access site induration or elevated white blood cells. The initial step is to draw two sets of blood cultures. The first should come from the dialysis catheter and the second from a peripheral site. Empiric intravenous antibiotics are indicated to cover gram-positive organisms until culture and sensitivities return. Furthermore, most dialysis catheters are in the internal jugular or subclavian veins with their tips lying near the right atrium. That leaves dialysis patients at risk for right-sided endocarditis. Thus, echocardiograms are indicated if a new regurgitant heart murmur is auscultated or with persistently positive blood cultures.

Interventions

Patient Pre-Assessment Prior to Initiation of Dialysis

Areas that need to be assessed during the patient's predialysis exam include the following:

- Fluid status (heart sounds, respiration rate, effort and breath sounds, IVD, presence or absence of edema)
- Weight
- Bowel regularity
- Sleep problems
- Pain
- Residual renal function
- Bleeding or bruising
- Blood pressure, sitting and standing
- Temperature, pulse and respiration (TPR) with apical/peripheral pulse assessment
- Skin color, temperature, integrity, turgor
- Vascular access patency, lack of infection or bleeding
- Additional physical and lab data evaluation for any necessary interventions or medications needed

Physical Exam Findings During Each Dialysis Session

The following physical exam findings should be noted during each dialysis session:

- Weight
- Blood pressure
- Temperature
- Pulse
- Respiratory rate
- Edema
- Assessing access site skin integrity, color and signs of inflammation
- Jugular vein distention
- Assessing access site integrity for thrills and bruits

Weighing Dialysis Patients

Patients are weighed before and after each dialysis session. Weight helps determine how much ultrafiltration the patient needs during dialysis. Weight is a good measure for fluid retention between dialysis sessions. Patients are advised to limit weight gain to one pound (0.5 kg) per day between dialysis. Post-dialysis weight is referred to as dry weight or the weight of the patient after fluid has been removed. Ideally, dialysis should leave the patient in a euvolemic state. Inadequate dialysis may leave patients hypervolemic and possibly hypertensive. Over adequate dialysis will leave patients hypovolemic and hypotensive.

Blood Pressure Measurement During Dialysis

Blood pressure measurement is extremely important during dialysis. Foremost, dialysis personnel are looking for extremes of pressure (high or low). Most commonly one will encounter low blood pressures. This is usually due to the removal of fluid during dialysis. However, low blood pressures can be indicative of more serious complications including sepsis. Hypotension is a contraindication to dialysis and treatment must be stopped if the systolic blood pressure falls below 80 mm Hg. Hypertension can be an indication of hypervolemia. The high pressure can tax the heart as well as other organs. Ideally, dialysis should leave the patient in a euvolemic and normotensive state.

Monitoring Nutritional Status

Nutritional status is monitored through two main methods:

- The physical exam should include height, weight, weight changes, triceps skinfold and arm circumference. Serial measurements are important to trend nutritional status. The triceps skinfold and arm circumference are important indicators of body fat and protein stores.
- The biochemical tests used include albumin, prealbumin, creatinine and cholesterol. Albumin is the best studied and correlates with nutritional status and mortality. Prealbumin has a shorter half-life and can be used to monitor more acute changes. Creatinine and cholesterol are surrogate markers for protein intake and should be used to monitor nutritional status as well.

Pediatric Monitoring During Hemodialysis

Pediatric monitoring during dialysis includes blood pressure. This does not differ from adult monitoring. However, in children weighing less than 20 kilograms monitoring heart rate and oxygenation is required. This is done to guard against hypotension from excess fluid removal. Other signs of hypotension include lethargy, yawning and irritability. Continuous monitoring in this patient population is necessary to record subtle changes in condition.

Items Necessary to Conduct a Predialysis Machine Assessment

Items necessary in dialyzer membrane check for patency and integrity:

- Blood tubing without leaks
- Accurate dialyzer
- Proper dialysate fluid composition
- Temperature limits
- Conductivity
- Extracorporeal blood circuit free of air
- Review of physician orders
- All alarms are programmed and functioning
- Dialysis water check for chloramines and other harmful agents

Parameters Monitored by Dialysis Machine

The dialysis machine monitors the following:

- Arterial pressure
- Venous pressure
- Fluid removal
- Dialysate flow
- Blood flow
- Heparin pump
- Air leak alarm
- Blood leak alarm

Calculating Transmembrane Pressures for Fluid Removal

The transmembrane pressure can be manually entered into the dialysis machine for ultrafiltration. Today, most machines will automatically calculate the transmembrane pressure. However, knowledge of how to ascertain the transmembrane pressure is important. The formula is as follows:

- Weight to be removed in milliliters + oral fluid intake during treatment + fluid to be removed from IV infusion during treatment = total fluid to be removed.
- Total fluid to be removed/number of hours on dialysis
- Total from previous step/kuf (coefficient of dialyzer) of dialyzer = transmembrane pressure

Venous Pressure

The venous pressure measures pressure in the line returning blood from the dialyzer to the patient. The venous pressure is monitored under preset parameters and alarms will sound if the pressures exceed those parameters. A sudden rise in venous pressure indicates an obstruction to flow via a clot or kink in the line. A sudden drop in venous pressure may indicate an arterial line clot or the venous needle was removed. Once activated, the alarm will halt dialysis until the problem is remedied.

Arterial Pressure

The arterial pressure does not refer to the patient's systemic blood pressure. Rather, this is the pressure measured in the arterial blood line leading towards the dialysis machine. The arterial pressure is a negative pressure. That means that the blood leaving the patient is being sucked out under negative pressure as it approaches the dialysis machine. The arterial pressure is monitored with an alarm under preset ranges. A suddenly high arterial pressure is indicative of some obstruction to flow (usually a clot or kink in the line). The alarm will sound and blood flow will cease until the problem is remedied.

Appropriate History Elicited from Patients in Preparation for Access

All patients should be asked the following:

- Have you previously had a central venous catheter?
- Which is the dominant arm?
- Do you have a pacemaker?
- Do you have congestive heart failure?
- Did you recently have a large peripheral or intravenous catheter?
- Are you on anticoagulation?
- Do you have a history of valvular heart disease or valve replacement?
- Do you have a history of neck, arm or chest surgery or trauma?
- Do you have any history of failed access?

The following is a list of the clinical relevance from each of the history questions asked of patients prior to access:

- Dominant arm—Attempt to use non-dominant arm for access
- Pacemaker—Associated with central vein stenosis
- Congestive heart failure—Access can exacerbate CHF via high output cardiac failure
- Recent peripheral access—The integrity of the vein will be damaged and time is required to allow for vessel healing
- Anticoagulation—Can be a contraindication since frequent venous and arterial punctures are required
- Valvular heart disease or replacement—Access increases susceptibility of cardiac valve infections
- History of neck, arm, chest trauma/surgery—Vessel damage limits access options
- History of failed access—Limits sites where access is available

Appropriate Timing and Precautions to Prepare Patients for Vascular Access

Patients with chronic kidney disease stage IV and V should be made aware of their prognosis and need for renal replacement. Consent must be obtained and type of access discussed with the patient. In general, fistulas require 6 months lead time prior to dialysis, arterio-venous grafts require 3-6 weeks, peritoneal catheters need 2 weeks and permcaths can be used immediately. In preparation for permanent access, the upper extremity should not be punctured with small intravenous lines, peripheral intravenous central catheters (PICC) or subclavian catheters. This helps ensure the integrity of the native veins and arteries in preparation for fistulas and grafts.

Assessing the Internal Access Point

The proper techniques that are recommended for assessing the internal access point before inserting the needle are as follows:

- Assess the proposed site before cleaning it.
- Observe for signs of infection: redness, inflammation, or warmth. Cold could indicate thrombosis. Check prior injection sites for healing, scabbing, and open sores. Assess for bruising, pain, numbness, or edema. If swelling is present, the circumference of the circumference should be tape-measured for later comparison to assess the progress.
- Palpate the internal access for the "thrill", a gentle vibration, which should be present over the total length. A pulse indicates less than adequate blood flow. Listen with the bell of a stethoscope for the sound of a swooshing sound, or bruit. If the bruit, swoosh and thrill are absent, the access may be clotted and should not be used.

PLACEMENT OF DIALYSIS NEEDLES

The steps used to govern the proper placement of the dialysis needles are as follows:

- The venous needle must always be placed in the same direction of the blood flow (also known as antegrade).
- The arterial needle is nearest the anastomoses (but at least 3 cm away from the site to avoid its cannulation).
- The arterial needle may be antegrade or retrograde (away from the heart).
- The venous needle must be at least 5 cm proximal to the arterial needle.
- Since the AV fistula and AV graft are cannulated at different angles, adjust insertion angle (from 20-45°) to accommodate for these differences.
- New AV fistulas are fragile and must be approached with care, usually by highly experienced personnel. It may initially be cannulated with one needle-arterial outflow, and the venous return may be accomplished by use of a central venous catheter.

NEEDLE POSITIONING

Needle positioning is important for many reasons. The placement of needles for dialysis should be done only after these facts are considered:

- There are potential problems with inadequate long-term patency rate of the access.
- Aneurysms may development from placing the needles in the same place, which affects vessel walls by making them become thin.
- Needle sites must be rotated to avoid this weakening of vessel walls.
- Placing the arterial needle near the anastomoses achieves optimal blood flow.
- The needle tip should remain more than 3 cm away from anastomoses.
- The usual practice is to place the arterial needle with the flow.
- Spacing needles 5cm apart minimizes recirculation of the blood, which could lead to inadequate dialysis.

BUTTONHOLE TECHNIQUE OF ACCESSING A VASCULAR ACCESS POINT

The buttonhole technique is a constant site technique in which an AV fistula is accessed for cannulation through the exact same site and at the same angle, creating a tunnel tract of scar tissue. This tract allows for easier cannulation, using the same scarred channel each time. This results in less pain for the patient and fewer cases of infiltration and may be a helpful alternative for the patient who dialyzes at home. Medisystems has a dull needle for use once the buttonhole is fully developed; this prevents the patient from cutting the tissue encircling the tunnel track.

PREFERRED ACCESS TYPES

According to the National Kidney Foundation, access types should be in the following order of preference:

9. Fistulae are preferred in the following order:
   a. Wrist (radiocephalic) primary fistula
   b. Elbow (brachiocephalic) primary fistula
   c. Transposed brachial basilic vein
10. Arterio-venous grafts are less preferred than fistulae. They should be placed at the following locations in descending order:
    a. Forearm
    b. Upper arm
    c. Chest wall or lower extremity

11. Long-term catheters should be generally avoided. In order of descending preference:
    a. Long term (tunnel cuffed) catheters
    b. Short term catheters

AV GRAFT

Arteriovenous grafts are a conduit between arteries and veins. A synthetic (most common) or biocompatible conduit is inserted subcutaneously connecting an artery with a vein. Blood flows from the artery into the graft and empties in the vein. The graft requires 2-6 weeks to mature. It is important to note the direction of blood flow. Blood returning from the hemodialysis machine must enter the venous line and flow in the same direction as arterial blood. This will ensure that venous resistance is not high and that physiologic flow in the body is maintained without too much turbulence. It will also help prevent recirculation (already dialyzed blood returning to the dialyzer).

ADVANTAGES OF ARTERIO-VENOUS GRAFTS

AV grafts have the following advantages:

- Large vessel for easier access during dialysis
- Shorter time to maturation for use (3-6 weeks)
- Many insertion sites
- Technically easier for surgeons
- Easy to repair

NORMAL PHYSICAL FINDINGS FOR AV GRAFTS

The normal physical findings for AV grafts include:

- No irregular areas or sites of aneurysms
- Low pitch systolic and diastolic sounds
- Thrill palpated best at the arterial anastomosis but also throughout the graft with easy compressibility

ARTERIOVENOUS FISTULA

Fistulae are created by vascular surgeons. Small incisions are made in the forearm or elbow and an adjoining artery and vein is anastomosed. The increased blood flow from the artery into the vein causes venous dilation. The vein must be allowed to fully dilate and mature which is about a six-month process. Fistulae are the most preferred method for hemodialysis access because of their decreased infection and clotting rates. The procedure is usually done in an office setting and is relatively quick. Arm exercises are also prescribed to the patient to help facilitate fistula maturation.

NORMAL PHYSICAL FINDINGS FOR AV FISTULAE

The normal physical findings for fistulae include:

- Well developed venous outflow with no areas of aneurysms
- The vessels partially collapse when the patient raises his/her arm above head
- Low pitch diastolic and systolic murmur with auscultation
- Thrill felt best at the arterial site but can be felt throughout the entire outflow vein

NEEDLES USED FOR PUNCTURING THE AV FISTULA

The preferred type of needle that is used to accommodate high blood flows in high-flux or high-efficiency dialyzers have the following features:

- The preferred needle type has a large gauge, which allows for high blood flows, high-flux, or high-efficiency dialysis. Blood flows of 400-500 mL/min with 14-gauge needles, 17- gauge are used in children and infants, although it is recommended to use at least a 15-gauge, which accommodates a large volume of blood flow of 350 mL/min or more. Dialyzing with a small gauge needle may cause hemolysis of red-blood cells due to the cells passing through the needle with such force that they are ruptured.
- The preferred needle type has a thin-wall.
- The preferred needle type has a back-eye.

ADVANTAGES OF FISTULAE OVER OTHER ACCESS TYPES

Fistulae are recommended by the National Kidney Foundation because of their lower complication rates. Foremost, they have the lowest rate of thrombosis and failures. Thus, they require fewer interventions, which make them very cost effective. Fistulae do not get infected as often as permcaths or grafts. The combination of the stated advantages leads to lower hospitalizations and increased survival for dialysis patients.

WRIST AND ELBOW FISTULAE

The wrist and elbow offer the following advantages:

- Greater patency to flow after maturing
- Lower rates of stenosis, infection and vascular steal (the new conduit "steals" blood from the radial artery).

The disadvantages include:

- Long time to mature (usually 1 – 4 months)
- Difficulty accessing the vein during dialysis relative to grafts
- Cosmetically displeasing

The wrist is the first choice by surgeons in choosing access sites. The reasons include:

- Technically easy site to work with
- Preserves proximal vessels in case the fistula fails
- Fewer adverse events including thrombosis, infections and vascular steal.

The major disadvantage to wrist fistulae is that it offers a lower blood flow rate in comparison to more proximal, larger vessels. The elbow is the second choice for fistulae behind the wrist.

The major advantages include:

- Higher blood flow rate
- Easier to cannulate for hemodialysis access (large vessel)

The disadvantages include:

- Technically more difficult for surgeons
- More edema
- Higher incidence of vascular steal and stenosis

CANNULATING A MATURE FISTULA OR GRAFT

The following is the proper technique for cannulating a mature fistula or graft:

- First, the skin is prepped with proper infection control techniques.
- A tourniquet must be applied proximal to the fistula. This will decrease venous return and help engorge the fistula for easier access.
- Then pull the skin in the opposite direction from needle insertion.
- For arterial puncture, the needle can be either in the same or opposite direction as blood flow.
- For venous punctures, the needle must be inserted in the same direction as blood flow.
- After inserting the needle, it should be advanced slowly and taped to the skin surface.
- Once dialysis is over the needle should be removed at the same angle as it was inserted (this prevents vessel tearing).
- Pressure should not be applied to the needle site until after it is removed (to avoid vessel trauma and blood splashes).

FISTULA AND GRAFT SURVEILLANCE OF PATENCY

It is important to monitor patency of both fistulae and grafts to ensure adequate dialysis and continued access. The National Kidney Foundation lists the following techniques as preferred or acceptable means of monitoring access patency:

- Doppler ultrasound
- Magnetic resonance angiography (MRA)
- Various dilution techniques
- Physical findings

The physical findings include loss of palpable thrill, lack of bruit on auscultation, persistent arm swelling, presence of collateral veins and prolonged bleeding.

MONITORING, SURVEILLANCE AND DIAGNOSTIC TESTING AS RELATED TO VASCULAR ACCESS

Monitoring refers to the examination and evaluation of the vascular access via physical examination to detect physical signs that suggest the presence of dysfunction. Surveillance is the periodic evaluation of the vascular access by using tests that may involve special instrumentation and for which an abnormal test result suggests the presence of dysfunction. Diagnostic testing refers to specialized testing that is prompted by some abnormality or other medical indication and that is undertaken to diagnose the cause of the vascular access dysfunction.

PREFERENCE OF FISTULAE AND GRAFTS OVER LONG-TERM CATHETERS

Long-term catheters (permcaths) are associated with high infection rates and are frequently clotted. Furthermore, a permcath placed in the subclavian or internal jugular veins drains near the right atrium. This will subject the patient's cardiac valves (particularly tricuspid) to infections by staphylococcus and streptococcus. Fistulae and grafts also last longer, decrease hospitalizations, and improve patients' quality of life. All long-term catheters should be placed with plans for more permanent access.

Dialysis Catheter

The use of the central venous catheter may result in subclavian vein stenosis; therefore, it should only be chosen as a temporary alternative to traditional modes of hemodialysis. The situations that would indicate the use of a dialysis catheter in a hemodialysis patient are as follows:

- When the need arises for acute dialysis access, before mature access
- For the patient with an imminent kidney transplantation surgery
- When awaiting the AV access maturation
- When the availability of appropriate vessels is limited for permanent internal access
- For the patient receiving plasmapheresis
- For patient receiving venovenous continuous renal replacement therapy
- For patient with peritonitis who usually use peritoneal dialyses
- For patients who have acute overdose or intoxication

Catheter Types

Different types of catheters used for dialysis include the following:

- Cuffed and uncuffed: Uncuffed catheters when used over a prolonged period are often associated with a high infection rate. Cuffed are preferable due to their Dacron or felt cuffs, which reduce the incidence of infection and catheter migration.
- Dual-lumen catheters in a side-by-side (double-D) configuration result in less recirculation and have a larger separation of inlet and outlet ports and more pliable catheters.
- The palindrome symmetrical tip reduces recirculation.
- The Tesio catheter system features 2 separate catheters, one for inflow and one for outflow, made of softer silicone material.

Veins Chosen for Temporary Vascular Access

Veins chosen for temporary vascular access are the subclavian, internal jugular, and femoral veins. Subclavian and jugular veins are used in certain patients, but for others these sites are contraindicated.

- Patients with difficulty breathing who cannot be placed in supine or Trendelenburg positions, and those with subclavian vein stenosis are not candidates for subclavian or jugular access.
- The right internal jugular is the optimal insertion site. The subclavian vein should not be used due to the complications that may result, including hemothorax, pneumothorax, subclavian artery perforation, brachial plexus injury, and a higher rate of venous stenosis. For short-term catheter placement, the femoral artery is a good choice. If a femoral catheter is used, it should be at least 20cm in length to assure that the tip is located in the inferior vena cava for good blood flow and to minimize recirculation.

Femoral Catheter

There are certain times that the use of a femoral catheter for dialysis is indicated. These are as follows:

- When an acutely ill patient is confined to bed
- When dialysis is needed immediately and the access is compromised as in the end stage renal disease (ESRD) patient
- For continuous renal replacement treatment
- When the patient has subclavian vein stenosis

Complications that may occur immediately after insertion of a catheter into the femoral vein are as follows:

- Pneumothorax
- Hemothorax
- Air embolism
- Bleeding from inadvertent puncture of femoral artery

INFECTION AT CATHETER SITE

One of the complications of catheter placement that may occur is infection. Signs and symptoms of infection at the catheter site include the following:

- Fever or chills
- Severe cases exhibit hemodynamic instability
- Septic symptoms

Causative agents are frequently Gram-positive organisms, usually of the Staphylococcus species, but Gram-negative may be associated with up to 40% of infections. Treatment begins with blood cultures and continues with administration of systemic antibiotics that cover both Gram-positive and Gram-negative bacteria. Vancomycin should be given a methicillin-resistant Staphylococcus has been detected in the dialysis population. Removal of the catheter is recommended. One week after the completion of antibiotic therapy, blood cultures should be repeated.

LIMITATIONS OF PLACING LONG-TERM CATHETERS

Permcaths should not be placed in the following two regions:

- Where current or future AV access is maturing or to be placed
- In femoral veins in patients waiting for transplants.

Arterio-venous fistulae need time to mature as do AV grafts. Thus, placing a permcath near the site of maturing or future access sites will endanger the fistula or graft. In patients on the transplant list, access via the femoral vein should be avoided. The reasoning includes placing the patient at risk for femoral vein thrombosis. The femoral vein is near the renal vein and anything that may compromise that vasculature should be avoided.

TUNNELED CUFFED CATHETERS

Tunneled cuffed catheters offer the following advantages:

- All patients can receive them
- Easily inserted at various sites
- Can be used immediately post insertion
- Skin puncture is not necessary
- No hemodynamic consequences, e.g. high output cardiac failure
- Low costs
- Can be used as short term brides until grafts and fistulae mature

The major disadvantages of tunneled catheters include:

- High rates of infection
- High rates of thrombosis
- Central venous stenosis

- Cosmetically displeasing
- Short shelf life
- Lower blood flow rates which increases dialysis times

LifeSite Hemodialysis Access System

The LifeSite Hemodialysis Access System refers to an implantable device that is used as a central venous blood access port for hemodialysis. The system is comprised of a 1.2-inch round, 0.5-inch high metal valve with a 25-inch cannula line. The valve is placed subcutaneously with the cannula extending into the subclavian or jugular vein. Two systems are placed in the patient for both the draw and return of blood. A specialized 14-gauge needle is inserted into the LifeSite valve; this opens the internal pinch clamp, allowing for the flow of blood. Removing the needle allows the clamp to close. After several cannulations into the valve, a tract or buttonhole is created between the skin and valve entrance. An antimicrobial solution is used to irrigate the pocket valve between treatments.

Contraindications and Possible Complications

Contraindications associated with using the LifeSite Hemodialysis Access System include the following:

- Positive blood cultures associated with recent infection
- Systemic or localized infection that does not respond to antibiotic therapy
- Lack of adequate tissue to support placement of the valve
- Confirmed or suspected allergy to components of the device

Possible complications of the LifeSite Hemodialysis Access System are as follows:

- Inadequate blood flow
- Bleeding or hematoma at injection site
- Cannulation problems
- Thrombosis
- Site infections
- Valve pocket or cannula tunnel infections
- Bacteremia or septicemia

Monitoring Hemoglobin Levels

The best time to draw hemoglobin and hematocrit levels is predialysis. While one could argue that a postdialysis measurement of hemoglobin would be more accurate because is approximates the patient's dry weight, most studies have only examined predialysis levels. Moreover, all of the guidelines for management of anemia in patients on hemodialysis are based on predialysis data. Therefore, it is accepted practice and by convention that one draws and interprets the predialysis hemoglobin/hematocrit.

Urea Reduction Ratio

The urea reduction ratio is the percentage of urea removed during dialysis. The postdialysis urea is subtracted from the predialysis urea to give the amount that was removed. This amount is then divided by the predialysis urea and multiplied by 100% to give the percentage removed:

$$(BUN_{pre} - BUN_{post})/BUN_{pre} \times 100\%$$

An adequate urea reduction ratio is 65%. The urea reduction ratio is another indicator of dialysis adequacy.

Drawing Predialysis BUN from Patients with AV Fistulas, Grafts, and Permcaths

In patients with AV fistulas or grafts, the predialysis BUN should be drawn prior to initiating hemodialysis. The sample should be taken from the arterial port. The syringe should be free of any saline or heparin so as not to dilute the sample. In patients with permcaths, the first 5 cc of blood should be drawn and discarded. This ensures that any remaining heparin or saline that remains in the catheter is discarded. Then the sample should be drawn and sent for analysis. Again, this should be done prior to the initiation of hemodialysis. The blood sample needs to be drawn under sterile technique.

Collecting Post Dialysis BUN Samples

Post dialysis BUN samples should be collected as follows:

- First, the dialysate flow should be stopped or decreased to the lowest permitted setting for 3 minutes.
- Then the blood flow rate should be decreased to 100 mL/min for 15 seconds. This prevents auto recirculation of blood from artificially diluting the BUN and falsely elevating Kt/V.
- After the 15 seconds, the blood pump should be stopped and the sample can be drawn under sterile technique. Blood should be obtained from either the arterial port side.

Again, waiting 15 seconds under the low flow rate is important to obtain an accurate post BUN sample.

Dialysis Adequacy

Dialysis adequacy is measured with the formula Kt/V. Kt/V is a complex formula that assesses how well each dialysis session went. The K represents a kinetic factor for urea, t is for dialysis time and v is a calculated guess at the volume of distribution for urea. Memorizing the exact calculations involved is not necessary but a pre- and post-dialysis BUN is required along with pre- and post-dialysis weights. The former is an indication of urea clearance and the latter for volume removed. Current guidelines suggest a Kt/V of greater than 1.2. A level of less than 1.2 indicates inadequate dialysis and is associated with worse outcomes. All dialysis centers keep track of Kt/V for all patients as a metric of quality control.

According to the National Kidney Foundation, dialysis adequacy can be adversely affected via three main categories:

12. compromised urea clearance
13. reduced treatment time
14. laboratory errors

Urea clearance can be compromised through the following:

- Access recirculation
- Inadequate blood flow from vascular access
- Inaccurate estimation of dialyzer performance
- Inadequate dialyzer reprocessing
- Clotted dialyzer fibers
- Errors in blood and dialysate flow rates caused by miscalibrated equipment
- Inadequate blood and dialysate flow rate
- Dialyzer leaks

Reduced treatment time can occur with early discontinuation of treatment, inaccurate time of dialysis recorded and not accounting for interruptions during dialysis treatments. Finally, laboratory errors occur with dilution of BUN blood samples, drawing pre and post dialysis BUN at the wrong time, laboratory errors and drawing post dialysis BUN after more than five minutes after the end of dialysis.

Education

PREDIALYSIS EDUCATION

The most important predialysis education goals include these:

- Supply information about preferred dialysis modalities
- Endorse home dialysis
- Encourage responsibility and self-reliance for personal health

When GFR is 20mL/min or the condition is rapidly declining, these procedures should be followed:

- Use written materials
- Encourage internet research
- Suggest group sessions
- Provide individual sessions with dialysis nurse

Group sessions should do the following:

- Allow time for patients to interact with others with similar health concerns
- Encourage discussion of dialysis modalities
- Invite current dialysis patients for personal insights

Individual sessions should follow these guidelines:

- Be scheduled after group sessions
- Respond to questions arising from group discussions
- Assess patient's comprehension of dialysis treatment alternatives
- Incorporate a visit to PD and HD training facilities and interactions with patients currently in training

CRITICAL SIGNS AND SYMPTOMS TO BE AWARE OF POST-DIALYSIS

Electrolyte abnormalities can develop following dialysis, with hyperkalemia being the most common. Symptoms the patient may experience with this include numbness or tingling and palpitations, though it is usually asymptomatic. Other electrolyte abnormalities that can occur include hyponatremia, hypocalcemia, and hypermagnesemia. Dialysis disequilibrium syndrome is common and is characterized by weakness, dizziness, and headache. Mental status changes can occur in severe cases. The patient should monitor their fistula site for any acute signs of infection. It should also be palpated for a thrill. The absence of a thrill may indicate a blood clot. Bleeding from a vascular access site may occur due to the heparin often used in dialysis to prevent clotting. This can usually be controlled with elevation and pressure at the site. Patients receiving peritoneal dialysis need to be alert for the signs of peritonitis, which include abdominal pain or a cloudy effluent. Peritonitis occurs approximately once per patient per year. Patients should also be aware of the common symptoms of anemia because this is common with kidney failure.

RENAL REPLACEMENT THERAPY MODALITIES

The patient needs to be made aware of all of the options available for the treatment of renal replacement therapy. These include the following:

- Pre-emptive kidney transplantation: survival superior to standard dialysis
- Dialysis, home vs. in-center therapy: availability in local area, transportation issues, status of patient's home, support structure, technical issues

- Short daily hemodialysis, 5 day a week treatments decrease cramping and hypotension
- Long nocturnal dialysis, 8-10 hours in length, usually done at home
- Peritoneal dialysis, decreases requirement for special water systems, simple equipment setup, better mobility
- Palliative care with no dialysis

METHODS OF MONITORING NUTRITIONAL STATUS

Other than serum laboratory tests and physical exams, methods of monitoring nutritional status include the following:

- Taking dietary history and keeping diaries
- Use of the subjective global assessment survey (a validated survey looking at patient's total well being)
- Protein catabolic rate (examines the difference between nitrogen intake and waste)
- Dual Energy X-ray Absorptiometry (DEXA) scans (whole body DEXA scans are a reliable way to examine body composition irrespective of fluid status)

DIETARY RESTRICTIONS IN PATIENTS WITH CHRONIC KIDNEY DISEASE STAGES II-IV

Patients with chronic kidney disease should adopt the following dietary habits:

- Low protein
- Low sodium
- Low phosphorus

The low protein diet is helpful in reducing the amount of nitrogenous waste produced with protein breakdown. Nitrogenous wastes help contribute towards uremia. A low phosphorus diet is also important to limit the amount of phosphorus absorption. Increased phosphorus coupled with calcium can lead to calcium-phosphate deposition into tissues causing damage and ischemia. Finally, limiting sodium intake is crucial to lowering blood pressure and decrease water retention. Hypertension is both a cause and a consequence of renal failure and sodium restriction has been implicated in causing and exacerbating high blood pressure.

DIETARY RESTRICTIONS ON POTASSIUM AND PHOSPHORUS IN PATIENTS ON DIALYSIS

Potassium should be limited to approximately 70 mEq/day. Multiple factors are involved in regulating potassium intake including size of the patient, dialysate used and medications. An excellent source (hazard) of potassium includes vegetables and fruits, particularly bananas. Phosphorus intake should be limited to 600 – 1200 mg/day. Phosphorus intake is largely controlled by phosphate binders and an excellent source of phosphorus includes protein and soda.

PROTEIN INTAKE REQUIREMENTS

Patients on hemodialysis should aim for a goal of 1.2 gm/kg of body weight per day. Patients on peritoneal dialysis should aim for a goal of 1.3 gm/kg of body weight per day. Patients on dialysis have higher protein requirements because they lose amino acids with each dialysis session. Moreover, malnutrition is a problem with dialysis patients and studies have shown that low albumin is correlated with increased hospitalizations. Proteins come from two sources: animal and plant.

- Animal sources include all essential amino acids and good choices include fish, chicken.
- Plant sources include legumes and nuts.

Water Intake

Water intake is largely contingent on urine formation plus insensible losses. The ability to closely match water intake with output will help with water homeostasis and maintain balance. Thus, water input is entirely patient specific. If, however, the patient does not make any urine then only insensible losses should be recovered. Excess water intake leads to hypertension exacerbation and left ventricular hypertrophy. Acceptable limits to weight gain between dialysis sessions is 1.5 kg.

Vitamin Supplementation and Trace Minerals

Vitamin supplementation may be necessary in patients on dialysis. Dialysis patients are at risk for vitamin deficiencies, particularly water-soluble vitamins. Supplementation with vitamins B1, B2, B6, B12 and niacin and folate is acceptable. Excess vitamins A and C should be avoided for they are toxic in renal patients. Trace minerals do not need to be replaced routinely. A daily multivitamin is more than enough to replace the needed minerals lost.

Providing Supplemental Nutrition

There are essentially three ways of supplying supplemental nutrition:

- Orally
- Intradialytic parenteral nutrition
- Intraperitoneal amino acid dialysate for peritoneal dialysis patients

Oral supplementation usually comes as protein shakes such as Ensure. Intradialytic parenteral nutrition (IDPN) is the administration of proteins and calories during dialysis. It is used in patients who cannot take or do not adequately respond to oral supplements. For peritoneal dialysis patients, intraperitoneal amino acid dialysate is used. Amino acids are substituted for a portion of the dextrose and have been shown to increase protein intake.

Dietary Differences Between Peritoneal Dialysis and Hemodialysis Patients

Peritoneal dialysis patients require some differences in dietary intake. Foremost, they require more protein due to the larger protein losses with peritoneal dialysis. The caloric intake is similar for both patients but the peritoneal patient absorbs more dextrose. The dextrose adds more calories and can exacerbate hypertriglyceridemia in obese diabetics or be helpful in undernourished patients. Sodium and fluid intake not need be as stringent as with hemodialysis patients. This is due to the ability of the dialysate to remove excess fluid with more frequent exchanges. Potassium is also less of a problem because of the infusion of insulin with each exchange. The insulin forces potassium into the cells and lowers serum K levels. However, phosphorus is more difficult to control in peritoneal dialysis patients. The phosphorus is usually accompanied with protein and thus more phosphate binders are required.

Medication Administration

Volume of Distribution

Volume of distribution refers to the volume of plasma required to maintain a certain concentration of a drug. It is defined by the equation:

Volume of distribution = Total amount of drug in the body/drug concentration.

The volume of distribution is not a real volume but an arbitrary value. Drugs that are absorbed into the blood are either protein bound or free. Because nly the free drug is active, a highly bound drug is said to have a small volume of distribution. In dialysis, increased fluid retention coupled with lower albumin (malnutrition) leads to increased volume of distribution. In addition, the increased serum acidity alters how albumin binds to medications, which often leads to a more free drug. Thus, most drugs need to be given at lower doses or with less frequency.

Bioavailability

Bioavailability refers to the amount of drug that is absorbed and becomes available for use. Bioavailability is largely contingent on route of administration, intrinsic characteristics of the drug and environmental factors. Drugs can be administered orally, subcutaneously, intramuscularly or intravenously, or can be inhaled. Each route will offer a different bioavailability. For example, an oral drug has to get absorbed from the gut and pass through the liver before being available for use while an intravenous medication is not subject to the gut or liver. Thus, for a given drug dosage the bioavailability of an intravenous administration is higher than oral. In dialysis patients, uremia alters the stomach pH (higher than normal). The lower acidity alters drug absorption. Other medications taken such as phosphate binders and H2 blockers also alter gut pH. Finally, uremia alters liver enzymatic activity. Some drugs are more available whereas others are less so.

Half-Life

Half-life is the amount of time needed for the body to eliminate 50% of a drug. This is an exponential decline in drug concentration and half-life is useful in helping one deduce how long a drug will remain active in the body. In dialysis patients, the half-life of medicines is increased. This is secondary to larger volumes of distribution and lower clearance rates.

Clearance

Clearance can be understood by the simple equation:

$$\text{clearance} = \text{rate of drug removal}/\text{concentration}.$$

Clearance is the volume of blood that is completely removed from a substance over time. However, clearance is not simply clearing the blood of a drug or toxin but rather how that substance is removed from the blood. For example, both urea and glucose are filtered at the glomerulus. Urea is cleared by the kidney at a rate of 65mL/min. In contrast, glucose is cleared by the kidney at 0 mL/min. That means that glucose is filtered by the kidney but is completely reabsorbed and thus its clearance is zero. Urea, on the other hand, is not completely reabsorbed and so its clearance is higher. In dialysis patients, the clearance for most drugs is lower. This is because not all drugs are dialyzable (only small molecular weight medicines are dialyzed). Clearance is useful in monitoring maintenance doses and in dialysis patients the doses are usually decreased.

Medications for ESRD Patients

Selection of a medication to treat an ESRD patient requires special consideration by the physician. The effects on kidney function, electrolyte balance, and uremia must be taken into account. Any agent that will cause an increase in the metabolite load or be a detriment to the disease state should be avoided. Any drug that increases levels of urea, sodium, potassium, or acids further stresses the already failing kidney. Nephrotoxic drugs should also be used with great care. If possible, a single drug that can treat multiple conditions is preferable over numerous agents.

Loading Dose and Maintenance Dose

"Loading dose" refers to the amount or dosage of a drug that must be administered in order to obtain a therapeutic plasma level as quickly as possible. Loading doses can be dangerous because of their rapid administration technique and the increase in the blood plasma level of the drug. Loading doses are found in the drug reference literature but are calculated as the product of the required plasma concentration level (blood level "Cp") and the volume of distribution of the medication. The formula is as follows:

$$\text{Loading dose (mg/kg)} = V_d \text{ (mL/kg)} \times Cp \text{ (mg/mL)}$$

Once this value is determined in mg/kg, multiply this dose by the patient's ideal weight.

NEED FOR ANTICOAGULATION DURING DIALYSIS

When blood comes into contact with dialyzers and tubing it tends to clot. The dialyzer and tubing are foreign substances that aid in clot formation. Moreover, access sites have a high tendency to clot. The order of clot formation in descending order is: catheter>graft>fistula. In order to prevent clots in either access or extracorporeal sites, anticoagulation is administered. The most commonly used anticoagulant is heparin. Heparin is well tolerated in dialysis patients because of its relatively short half-life. Also, should bleeding ensue an antidote is readily available to reverse heparin's affects (protamine sulfate).

ANTICOAGULATION IN PEDIATRIC HEMODIALYSIS

Anticoagulation in pediatrics is similar to that of adults. The heparin dose is weight based and thus both loading and maintenance doses are adjusted to the child's weight. The same goals of therapy hold. The activated clotting time should be approximately 1.5 times normal. However, neonates and children with little mass need tight controls of the adjusted clotting times. This particular population is subject to cerebral hemorrhage from heparin.

REGIONAL HEPARINIZATION

Regional heparinization refers to the continual infusion of heparin via the arterial line with a concurrent infusion of an antidote into the venous line before the blood is infused back into the patient. Trisodium citrate is used in the arterial line. Since a calcium-free dialysate must be used with trisodium citrate, calcium chloride must be added into the venous line to prevent blood returning to the patient with a low ionized calcium level. The major disadvantages of this type of heparinization are that numerous laboratory tests are required to assess the clotting time and calcium levels.

TIGHT HEPARINIZATION

"Tight heparinization" which is also known to as low-dose heparinization, refers to the technique of heparin administration in which the dosage is determined by frequent clotting times in order to maintain a clotting time of 90-120 seconds by ACT. This technique is often used for the patient's first dialysis treatment or for any patient at risk for bleeding, such as one who is menstruating, post surgery, or who has a central venous catheter that will be removed postdialysis. After the minimal priming dose is given, the usual dosage is 10 units/kg and is regulated to maintain an ACT of 110 ± 10 seconds.

ADMINISTRATION OF HEPARIN FOR DIALYSIS PATIENTS

Assuming the patient is not a risk for bleeding, there are two main methods of heparin administration. The first is called intermittent intravenous heparin technique. It involves a loading dose at the beginning of dialysis with intermittent, smaller doses later on. The goal of treatment is to keep the clotting time between 150 – 180 seconds (three times normal). The second technique is called continuous infusion which involves a loading dose of heparin given systemically. Heparin is then slowly given to the extracorporeal system only throughout dialysis. Clotting times are used to adjust heparin infusions.

Risks and Safe Administration

Heparin is an anticoagulant and thus places the patient at increased risk of bleeding. Patients who are at increased risk of bleeding should not receive heparin during dialysis. These include:

- Patients who are actively bleeding
- Have a clotting disorder
- Take anticoagulants
- Recent surgery
- Recent trauma
- Thrombocytopenia
- Allergic to heparin

Patients at increased bleeding risk should not receive heparin at all. Furthermore, dialysis patients have poorly functioning platelets and thus cannot easily form a clot to prevent bleeding. In order to safely administer heparin the following should be done:

- Base the heparin dose on the patient's dry weight
- Check clotting times every 30 minutes
- Check the dialyzer and tubing for evidence of clots
- Check the patient for evidence of ecchymosis
- Stop heparin 30 – 60 minutes before the completion of dialysis

Hemodialysis Done Without Heparinization

Hemodialysis done without the use of an anticoagulant is the therapy of choice for patients with an increased risk of bleeding, pericarditis, coagulopathy, or thrombocytopenia. The most common methods used are as follows:

- Bloodlines and dialyzer are primed with saline with 3000 units of heparin/L, and then this solution is discarded (this technique is not used for patients with extremely high risk of bleeding, such as liver disease).
- Blood flow rates are set as high as tolerated, 350-450 mL/min.
- The dialyzer is rinsed with 100-200 mL of saline as frequently as every 15 minutes up to once every hour, through the arterial line, and is inspected for clotting.

Reversing Drug-Induced Renal Damage

Drug-induced renal damage can often be reversed and further damage prevented if the following steps are taken:

- Discontinue nephrotoxic drug immediately.
- Administer saline intravenously to decrease nephrotoxins such as cyclosporine or cisplatin by dilution of the drugs in the renal tubules.
- Damage done by nonsteroidal anti-inflammatory agents (NSAIDS) may be diminished by administering misoprostol, a prostaglandin analog.
- Select drugs with the least probability of nephrotoxicity, such as acetaminophen, aspirin, nonacetylated salicylates, sulindac, or nabumetone.
- Give lowest effective dose of any drug for the shortest duration for effectiveness.

Psychological and Sociocultural Interventions

PSYCHOLOGICAL REACTIONS IN COPING WITH DIALYSIS

The most common reactions include:

- Anxiety—The most common initial reaction. Patients and their families are about to embark on a very new experience and significant life style changes are about to take place. Dialysis staff needs to be supportive.
- Depression—On the same spectrum as anxiety and the two emotions often coincide. Again, the uncertainty of life on dialysis along with life style changes leads to these feelings.
- Anger—Can be manifested in many ways. Often dialysis patients are frustrated with their disease but will express anger towards their family or staff.

In all three instances referral to a social worker or psychiatrist is important in helping patients and families cope.

PSYCHOLOGICAL STAGES OF ADJUSTMENT AFTER BEGINNING DIALYSIS

There are three stages of psychological adjustment once dialysis is started:

15. Honeymoon Period—When a patient first undergoes dialysis. This period usually lasts from 6 weeks to 6 months. The patient feels better about their prognosis and carries a positive outlook.
16. Period of Disenchantment and Discouragement—Patients experience a loss of hope and confidence. As they settle into life on dialysis, they begin to realize the restrictions it has on their lifestyle.
17. Period of Long-Term Adaptation—The patient begins to accept life with dialysis and all that it carries. Patients settle in to a routine with intermittent periods of depression.

STRESSORS EXPERIENCED BY ESRD PATIENTS

Dialysis patients often experience a variety of psychosocial stressors due to their chronic illness and time-consuming treatments. Some of the physical, psychological and psychiatric problem areas may include the following:

- Effects of the illness
- Dietary restrictions
- Scheduling constraints
- Fear of dying
- Marital discord, sexual dysfunction, hormonal effects
- Tense interpersonal relationships with family, medical staff, administrative personnel
- Expense of treatment
- Unemployment
- Psychological complaints, anxiety, anger, hostility and depression with feelings of lack of worth, lack of interest in daily activities, changes in weight, altered sleep patterns, fatigue, inability to concentrate and thoughts of suicide
- Psychiatric disorders such as dementia, delirium, psychosis, anxiety disorders, and drug abuse

DEPRESSION IN THE ESRD PATIENT

Treatment for depression in the dialysis patient may include drug therapy such as the following:

- Selective serotonin reuptake inhibitors (SSRIs) and tricyclic antidepressants (TCAs) must be taken for 4-6 weeks to see the effects.
- Selective norepinephrine reuptake inhibitors (SNRIs) must be used with caution in dialysis patients since they are excreted through the kidneys.
- Monoamine oxidase inhibitors (MAOIs) should be avoided due to potential for causing hypotension.

Nonpharmacologic options include the following:

- Psychotherapy (cognitive, behavioral, interpersonal, and supportive), group therapy or individual
- Electroconvulsive therapy, if no contraindications

Infection Control

HAND WASHING

Studies have shown that dirty hands are the number one reason for infections traveling from patient to patient, patient to staff, or staff to patient. Frequent hand washing with soap and water or with an alcohol-based cleanser is required. Moreover, anytime a health care provider travels from patient to patient, they should wash their hands.

STANDARD PRECAUTIONS IMPLEMENTED IN DIALYSIS UNITS

Standard precautions include the following:

- Barrier precautions which includes gloves, face shield masks and gowns
- Protection against sharps and needles (sharps container)
- Personal hygiene (hand washing)
- Avoidance of environmental contamination (no eating, drinking, smoking in the treatment room)

BARRIER PRECAUTIONS IN DIALYSIS CENTERS

The most commonly used barrier precautions include:

- Gloves
- Face shield masks
- Gowns

They are used to protect both patient and nurse from transmitted blood borne as well as other infectious agents. Gloves are to be worn whenever contacting blood, bodily fluids, mucous membranes or soiled products. Between patients, hand washing and glove changes are necessary. Face shield masks are used during any procedure when there is a risk of a blood splash. This includes cannulation of an AV graft or fistula as well as decannulation at the end of dialysis. Gowns should be worn to protect the body against blood splashes or bodily fluids coming in contact with the health care provider.

COMMON BLOOD BORNE PATHOGENS

The most common blood borne pathogens include:

- Hepatitis B
- Hepatitis C

- HIV, Hepatitis D
- Cytomegalovirus

The most commonly transmitted virus is Hepatitis B. All healthcare workers as well as dialysis patients should be immunized against Hepatitis B. Furthermore, immunization against Hepatitis B renders immunity against Hepatitis D. HIV transmission is also concerning but is not as easily transferable as Hepatitis B. In fact, the risk of acquiring HIV from a known HIV patient from a needle stick is 0.3%. Currently there is no vaccine against Hepatitis C. Cytomegalovirus is readily found in most people and is only an issue in the immunocompromised e.g. persons with HIV or on immunosuppressive therapy.

Prophylaxis in Staff after Accidental Needle Stick

In the event of a needle stick the most important thing is to thoroughly cleanse the wound. A thorough history from the patient is necessary. The main concern is for blood borne pathogens, specifically Hepatitis B, Hepatitis C and HIV. The following table describes what actions to take:

- Suspect Hepatitis B: If staff member is immune, check immune status. If staff member is unsure of immunity, check immune status and if okay then no further treatment. If staff member is not immune, give Anti-HB immunoglobulin and initiate vaccination.
- Suspect Hepatitis C: Check Hepatitis C viral RNA, anti-HCV antibodies and liver function tests at baseline and 4-6 weeks and 4-6 months. There is no current recommendation for prophylaxis.
- Suspect HIV: Give two or three drugs post exposure for prophylaxis treatment depending on risk factors of the source. Baseline, 6 weeks, 12 weeks and 6 months testing for HIV should be done.
- Patients are asked to get tested for the aforementioned viruses if they are unsure of their status. However, they are not obligated to consent for any of these tests.

Hepatitis B

Transmission

Hepatitis B is a DNA virus transmitted through the blood. It is commonly transmitted through needles, perinatally, sexually, nosocomially (in hospital and outpatient care facilities), or via transfusions and organ transplants. The rate of transmission from transfusions and organ transplant is lower with the advent of sensitive blood tests. Sexual transmission is the most common method of transference in the developed world. After inoculation with hepatitis B it is said to be an active infection. This is when the virus is most likely to be transmitted. Upon active infection, the body begins to mount an antibody response. Hepatitis B can be either cured or take on an active carrier state. The former is the most common but a few patients continue to carry hepatitis B. Chronic carriers are at increased risk of infecting others as well as developing liver cancer and cirrhosis. Hepatitis B is easily transmitted for the following two reasons:

- Each mL of blood contains millions of viral copies
- It can survive for days on inanimate objects such as counter tops, tubing, etc.

Precautions with Patients with Active Hepatitis B

Proper protocol for treating a patient with Hepatitis B:

- Patients with active Hepatitis B should be dialyzed in an isolation area.
- The area could be a separate room or one that is clearly demarcated with caution tape on the floor.
- A nurse dialyzing a Hepatitis B patient should not also dialyze a non-Hepatitis B patient during the same shift.

- Any time a health care worker enters or leaves the isolation area they must change gloves and gowns.
- Gloves and gowns are not permitted to leave the isolation area.
- Dialyzer reuse is never permitted on patients with Hepatitis B and there should be a dedicated Hepatitis B dialysis machine.

STAFF SCREENING

Screening for hepatitis B consists of either the HBsAG or anti-HBs blood tests. The former indicates infectivity and the latter indicates immunity. Healthcare workers that are vaccinated and have mounted a response do not need to be screened. Vaccinated healthcare workers who do not mount an adequate response need both HBsAG and anti-HBs every 6 months. Unvaccinated staff should also be screened every 6 months. However, the caveat is in those staff members who are positive for HBsAg or positive for Anti-HBs. The former only need annual HBsAg screening and the latter require no screening at all (they are immune by having recovered from the infection).

VACCINATION AND MONITORING

Hepatitis B is a three series vaccine that is given at baseline, one month and 6 months. There is no guarantee that all persons will mount an appropriate immune response. In these patients a booster vaccine is recommended. There are no recommendations for monitoring hepatitis B immunity after completing the series in health care workers. However, dialysis patients can lose immunity and thus yearly monitoring of Anti-HBs is recommended. If dialysis patients' immunity wane, a booster shot is necessary.

DIAGNOSING IMMUNITY IN PATIENTS OR STAFF WITH HEPATITIS B

Serum tests are routinely drawn in all health care workers and dialysis patients prior to initiating dialysis. The following blood tests are needed:

- HbsAG (hepatitis B surface antigen)
- Anti-HBc (antibodies against hepatitis B core antigen)
- Anti-HBs (antibodies against hepatitis B surface antigen)

The HBsAG indicates the patient or staff member has active Hepatitis B. Anti-HBs alone indicates immunity against Hepatitis B via vaccination. Anti-HBc along with Anti-HBs indicates that the patient had hepatitis B, have recovered, and are now immune. Patients who are positive for HBsAG are highly infective and must be dialyzed in isolation. Staff and patients with Anti-HBs are immune to hepatitis B and are permitted to work in the isolation area.

HEPATITIS C

Hepatitis C used to be known as non-A, non-B hepatitis prior to its discovery. It is an RNA virus that has no present cure. It is transmitted via the blood and is most commonly found in current or ex-intravenous drug users. Other methods of transmission include tattoos and multiple piercings. It is currently treated with interferon and ribavirin. Hepatitis C can cause fulminant hepatic failure early (rare) or liver failure after 20-40 years. It also increases the risk of liver cancer.

HIV

Human Immunodeficiency Virus (HIV) is an RNA virus transmitted via the blood or sexually. It has no cure and vaccines are not available to date. However, progress in highly active antiretroviral therapy (HAART) has made HIV a chronic disease. Patients are surviving in excess of twenty years because of HAART. HIV acts by attacking the body's immune system. Eventually, the immune system becomes so weakened that it cannot fight off the simplest infections or colds. It is also associated with a host of other morbidities. HIV is not easily transmissible. For example, a simple needle stick from a known HIV source carries a 0.3% transmission rate. Factors that increase the chances of transmission include: large bore needle, depth of invasion, and contact of the needle with blood from the source.

TUBERCULOSIS

Tuberculosis (TB) is a bacterium that commonly affects the lungs. While TB can be found in organs outside the pulmonary arena, it is most infective when it attacks the lungs. Transmission of tuberculosis is via respiratory droplets but very difficult. It requires prolonged, intimate exposure to acquire TB (e.g. on a long plane ride, nursing homes, prisons). Dialysis patients are immunocompromised because of their disease. Furthermore, they spend a lot of time in the dialysis center. Thus, TB can be easily transmitted from one patient to another or to staff. Current treatment for TB includes a four-drug regimen which must be taken for two months. The four drugs are isoniazid, rifampin, ethambutol and pyrazinamide. After two months, only isoniazid and rifampin are needed for an additional four months. Choice of drug therapy is dependent on culture sensitivity and local resistance rates.

Tuberculosis screening is done via yearly skin tests. A tuberculin skin test or PPD is placed subdermally and the induration read after 48 hours. Health care workers and dialysis patients have a positive PPD if the induration is greater than 10 mm. If a PPD is positive, a chest x-ray is ordered. A patient with a negative chest x-ray should receive isoniazid prophylaxis for 9 months. A patient with a positive chest x-ray should be treated for active tuberculosis. Patients with active tuberculosis can be dialyzed in respiratory isolation under negative pressure. All staff is required to wear masks prior to entering the isolation room.

MULTIDRUG RESISTANT *KLEBSIELLA* AND *ACINETOBACTER*

Multidrug resistant *Klebsiella* and *Acinetobacter* are also highly resistant gram-negative bacteria. The former is becoming increasingly common in patients with repeated infections following multiple courses of antibiotics. *Acinetobacter* is always an issue for it is difficult to treat regardless of how resistant it may be. Again, patients with these infections require standard precautions and infecting other patients is worrisome.

MRSA AND VRE

MRSA and VRE are resistant bacteria to methicillin and vancomycin respectively. Their incidence is increasing and proper barrier protection is warranted to prevent further transmission. Their impact on dialysis patients and staff includes the risk of transmitting resistant bacteria to other patients. Furthermore, they are difficult to treat and thus an outbreak could be disastrous. Patients with MRSA and VRE do not need isolation and standard precautions suffice.

PREPARING SKIN FOR CANNULATION OF GRAFT OR FISTULA

Described below is the proper preparation of the skin prior to cannulation of the graft or fistula:

- The skin should be palpated for the thrill of the graft or fistula. This is where the needle will be inserted.
- Next, the site is to be washed with either a combination alcohol/chorhexidine gluconate solution or alcohol/povidone solution.
- If either the patient or staff accidentally touches the insertion site after the alcohol preparation, the site is considered contaminated and must be rewashed.
- Clean gloves must be worn by staff throughout the entire process. If the gloves become contaminated at any time, they must be changed prior to cannulation.
- Finally, after cannulation new gloves must be worn between patients.

Infection Control Techniques Used on All Catheters

According to the National Kidney Foundation, the following guidelines should be used to lower infection rates:

- The catheter port site should be inspected for signs of infection prior to use before every dialysis session.
- The catheter dressing should be changed with new gauze after each session aseptic techniques must be used which involves the use of gloves for handling of all catheter related procedures and wearing of surgical masks by staff.

Signs of Infections or Vascular Steal Phenomena in Patients with Fistulae and AV Grafts

Signs of infection include erythema, swelling, induration, warmth and broken skin. This is usually indicative of a local cellulitis but systemic bacteremia must also be ruled out. Thus, two sets of blood cultures must be sent and intravenous antibiotics covering staphylococcus and streptococcus species begun (usually vancomycin). Alternate access must also be used while the infection resolves. Signs of vascular steal include the following: cool extremity with discoloration and nail bed changes. One should also compare the extremities for warmth, skin color changes and muscle strength. If the site of access differs from the other extremity, vascular steal should be ruled out.

OSHA Guidelines for Working with Chemical Disinfectants

OSHA guidelines for personnel safety when using chemical disinfectants include the following:

- Protective gear (eye shields, gloves, and waterproof gowns) should be worn.
- Sufficient ventilation is necessary.
- Splashes on skin or in eyes must be flushed immediately with copious amount of water and medical attention sought.
- A shower and eyewash station must be available.
- All personnel must be well-informed about these hazardous chemicals and their toxicity.
- Printed OSHA requirements and regulations must be available in every dialysis facility.
- Safety Data Sheets (SDS) must be accessible to staff at all times.
- Facility must maintain education records and health monitoring records for all employees.

Dialyzer Reprocessing

Reprocessing a dialyzer affects its ability to remove large solutes. Disinfectants that are usually used for dialyzer reprocessing include the following:

- Formaldehyde: second most commonly used disinfectant
- Glutaraldehyde: used in some facilities
- Heat: used in some facilities
- Bleach: decreases membrane clearance of large solutes
- Renalin: used in approximately 70% of facilities to decrease membrane clearance of large solutes such as β2-microglobulin (most commonly used disinfectant)

The labeling requirements are as follows:

- Patient's name: must be used for only one patient
- Number of prior uses
- Date of last reprocessing

- Social security number or birth date
- Additional warning label to notify staff of reuse status of dialyzer-not required, but recommended

Renalin

Either Renalin or formaldehyde is the product of choice most often used for the decontamination process for dialyzers. Renalin is a combination of peracetic acid, acetic acid, and hydrogen peroxide. A 0.5% solution of Renalin is required for disinfecting dialyzers, and it must remain in use for 11 hours. Aqueous formaldehyde (formalin) in a 4% solution must be used for 24 hours at room temperature in order to kill all microorganisms, including viruses and spores. A 1.5% formalin solution must be used at 100° F for a 24-hour period.

Formaldehyde

Potential Hazards

Formaldehyde (formalin) is a powerful chemical disinfectant. Formaldehyde (formalin) has been linked to nasal and lung cancer. Airborne concentrates as low as 0.1 parts per million may elicit an irritation response in the nose, eyes, and throat, as well as allergic reactions such as wheezing, cough, and asthma-related symptoms. Whenever this product is used, the air quality must be monitored. The OSHA standard for short-term exposure limit (STEL) is 2 ppm during a 15-minute period. Respiratory training is mandatory for personnel who work with reuse of dialyzers, and they must be fitted for respirators. Annual safety training is required for staff members who use these chemicals.

Formaldehyde Exposure

It is critical that the symptoms of formaldehyde reaction are recognized early. If formaldehyde has not been completely removed from the dialyzer, the patient may experience the following:

- Anxiety
- Bitter, peppery taste in mouth
- Burning at the venous needle site
- Numbness around the lips and mouth
- Chest pain
- Back pain
- Shortness of breath

Treatment for formaldehyde reactions are as follows:

- Immediately stop dialysis as hemolysis of red blood cells may occur.
- Remove approximately 10 mL of blood from each needle to ensure the cessation of formaldehyde infusion.

Topical Antiseptics

Topical antiseptics are used to clean the skin prior to inserting the cannulation needles. The topical antiseptic solutions most commonly used prior to the insertion of cannulation needles are povidone-iodine and isopropyl alcohol. To cleanse the skin over the proposed injection site, apply the antiseptic with a sterile gauze pad in a circular motion beginning at the proposed site, circling outward until the area cleaned is about 2 inches in diameter. If using the povidone-iodine, allow it to dry before inserting the needle. If isopropyl alcohol is used, insert the needle before the alcohol dries. Follow each manufacturer's instructions for each type of disinfectant to assure effective disinfection.

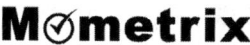

Governing Bodies That Establish Standards of Care for Dialysis Centers

The Joint Commission on accreditation of Healthcare Organizations (JCAHO) is an independent commission that establishes guidelines for standards of care for all dialysis facilities. Being subject to JCAHO inspections and receiving accreditation is essential for dialysis centers to remain open and for reimbursement from Centers for Medicare and Medicaid Services (CMS). Finally, CMS and state laws also play a role in establishing health care guidelines as well as water supply maintenance and cleanliness.

Patient Rights and Regulatory Guidelines

Dialysis Facility Structure

A typical dialysis facility is headed by a Director. This person is usually a nephrologist, albeit a multidisciplinary approach is taken. The nephrologist is chiefly involved with managing dialysis patients' renal disease and is responsible for writing dialysis orders. The dialysis nurse is the person responsible for the direct care of patients. They operate and manage the dialysis treatment, administer medications and collect blood samples for pre and post-dialysis values. Frequently, there is a nurse manager or nurse practitioner who oversees the nursing staff. Their main function is to work with nephrologists, nurses and other members of the team to help coordinate and facilitate care. Some dialysis centers also employ a dialysis technician. They are involved with dialysis equipment setup and maintenance. Finally, renal dietitians and social workers round up the major players in dialysis care. Dietitians help patients and their families organize renal responsive diets with particular attention to ensuring this population is not malnourished. Social workers aid patients and their families deal with psychological and other ethical issues.

HIPAA

HIPAA stands for health insurance portability and accountability act. This act was passed in 1996. It ensures patient privacy. All medical records and access to those records are available to health care professionals only. Moreover, the health care professional must access those records only in the interest of caring for the patient. If the health care worker is not actively caring for the patient, it is a HIPAA violation to access that patient's medical record. Furthermore, the sharing of medical information between health care personnel in a manner not specifically aimed at patient care (e.g. water cooler discussion) is prohibited. The information protected includes all information contained in paper charts, electronic medical records, laboratory results or oral communication.

Rights of Patient Prior to and After Beginning Hemodialysis

Foremost, patients have the right to decline dialysis provided a clinician has illustrated to them the risks, benefits and alternatives to refusing treatment. Patients must also consent prior to beginning any dialysis treatment, including transferring from one facility to another. Other patient rights include:

- To be informed about their disease and prognosis
- To be informed about the risks of treatment as well as the risks of withholding treatment
- To be informed about alternatives to treatment,
- To have the final say regarding their choice of treatment

Advance Directive

An advanced directive is a written document outlining the type of treatment a patient would want to receive should they lose the capacity to make decisions. An advanced directive can be as detailed as denying CPR or intubation or as general as assigning a health care proxy. A health care proxy can be anyone the patient assigns. The proxy is allowed to make treatment decisions for the patient as long as the patient does not have capacity. The proxy cannot make decisions which are contrary to the patient's wishes or written directive.

Process, Standard, and Clinical Indicator

The terms outlined are defined below:

- Process—A flow of procedures in carrying out an activity. For example, in order to prepare a patient for dialysis one needs the orders, proper dialysate, predialysis checking of the machine, dialyzer, etc. This is a process to get the patient ready for dialysis.
- Standards—Minimum parameters set by governing bodies to which all personnel are held accountable. For example, the American Nephrology Nurses Association sets standards for specific patient outcomes such as how to properly cannulate a graft or fistula.
- Clinical indicator—Measures used to evaluate patient outcomes. These are metrics outlined by governing bodies such as JCAHO. An example would be how many venous punctures are used to cannulate a graft or fistula.

KDOQI

The National Kidney Foundation has launched the Kidney Disease Outcomes Quality Initiative (KDOQI). It provides evidence-based guidelines for all dialysis personnel for all stages of chronic kidney disease. This initiative was first launched in 1997 and has ongoing research projects and recommendations for all to use. Currently, the National Kidney Foundation has 11 KDOQI guidelines and it is accepted practice to adhere to these guidelines.

CQI and TQM

CQI stands for continuous quality improvement. It operates under the umbrella of total quality management (TQM). CQI is an ongoing active process in which dialysis centers ask the following: how can we improve patient care? CQI implicates all types of quality outcomes from disease specific to dialysis procedure specific. The key to CQI is to keep it patient focused. CQI operates under TQM. TQM is upper management's commitment towards improving dialysis care and quality. Initiatives to improve care include vaccinations, infection rates, water quality control, etc.

Benchmark and Outcome

A benchmark provides a reference point for dialysis facilities. A benchmark could be national or local. For example, how does dialysis facility A compare with dialysis facility B in total mortality or infection rates? Benchmarks are useful in comparing how one is doing relative to others. An outcome is a clinically relevant metric used after some action has taken place. For example, a dialysis facility may decide to lower the number of infection rates by 50% by implementing new infection control guidelines. After implementing the guidelines, the infection rate is measured and compared to prior values.

Professional Boundaries

Professional boundaries must be maintained between healthcare workers and dialysis patients. "Professional boundaries" refer to the self-imposed restraints that the dialysis staff must maintain in order to achieve a therapeutic relationship with their patients. The National Council of State Boards of Nursing, Inc. defines this as "the spaces between the nurse's power and the client's vulnerability". Since dialysis patients may be under the care of the dialysis staff several times a week over a period of several years, a close relationship may develop. The healthcare worker should not overstep these boundaries by spending time with the patient after normal working hours, entering any business arrangements, socializing, having any sexual relationship, or accepting gifts or any type from the patient or family members. Intimate relationship with a patient is considered misconduct and a serious violation of the Nurse Practice Acts in most states.

Peritoneal Dialysis

ADVANTAGES AND DISADVANTAGES OF HD AND PD FOR THE ESRD PATIENT WITH DIABETES

The diabetic patient who undergoes in-center HD treatment has these advantages:

- Frequent medical observation
- Less loss of protein during dialysis treatment

The disadvantages are as follows:

- Higher risk of vascular access complications
- Risk of predialysis hyperkalemia
- Increase chance of hypotension during treatment

The advantages for the diabetic patient who chooses PD are as follows:

- Better glycemic control, especially with intraperitoneal insulin
- Better cardiovascular tolerance
- Better potassium control
- Vascular access is not required

The disadvantages are as follows:

- Peritonitis
- Protein loss
- Increase in intraabdominal pressure complications, for example gastroparesis

PERITONEAL DIALYSIS

Peritoneal dialysis uses the peritoneal cavity, which is approximately equal to the body's surface area, as a reservoir in which the dialysate is infused via a catheter. The peritoneum acts as a semipermeable membrane through which surplus body fluid and solutes, including uremic toxins, are removed (ultrafiltrate).

Peritoneal dialysis is the process by which dialysis can occur using the peritoneal membrane. Hypertonic dialysate filled with dextrose is infused into the peritoneum via an indwelling catheter. The dialysate fills the abdominal cavity. The peritoneum serves as the semipermeable membrane allowing for urea, potassium and other toxins to diffuse into the dialysate. Moreover, the dialysate is hypertonic which permits excess body water to diffuse into the peritoneum (ultrafiltration). The fluid is then drained and this entire process is known as an exchange.

Peritoneal dialysis allows the patient a simpler, home-based therapy with little need for special water systems. The equipment is easy to set up and use. The two types of PD are continuous ambulatory peritoneal dialysis (CAPD) where the patient performs manual exchanges 4-5 times a day and continuous cycling peritoneal dialysis (CCPD) where the exchanges are done while the patient is sleeping.

Patients who often favor PD include the following:

- Children and infants
- Patients with severe cardiovascular disease
- Patients with diabetes

- Patients who prefer the freedom
- Patients who prefer home dialysis, but have no one to assist them

DISADVANTAGES

While peritoneal dialysis offers patients the advantage of at home dialysis, it does come with some disadvantages. The first is an increase in malnutrition. The peritoneal membrane with frequent exchanges allows for excess protein loss. Protein malnutrition is very common in these patients. Moreover, the dextrose in the dialysate is reabsorbed. The dextrose causes hypertriglyceridemia and worsens obesity and diabetes. Finally, adequacy of dialysis is not as good when compared to hemodialysis. In order to comply with the K/DOQI guidelines for adequacy, patients are often asked to perform more exchanges with larger volumes each day.

ADVANTAGES FOR ELDERLY PATIENTS

The advantages of PD for the elderly patient consist of the following:

- No time, effort, or expense invested in traveling to the dialysis center
- Maintenance of control of their therapy, which promotes independence
- Preservation of usual lifestyle
- Ability to set own schedule
- Lack of need for vascular access, which is important because many elderly patients have poor peripheral vessels
- Maintenance of therapies, blood chemistry levels, and fluid status
- Slow, continuous therapy possible, preferable for correction of brain electrophysiologic and cognitive function abnormalities
- Less rigid dietary and fluid restrictions

DISADVANTAGES FOR ELDERLY PATIENTS

Some of the disadvantages of using PD as the mode of choice for the elderly patient include the following:

- The incidence of complications, such as dementia, hernias, peritonitis, *Staphylococcus epidermis*, and abdominal and catheter leaks all are higher in the elderly population on PD.
- If patient needs significant ultrafiltration, the dialysate glucose concentration may depress the appetite and lead to malnutrition even if dry weight is stable; dextrose provides calories but little nutrition (this may be hard to diagnose initially).
- There is a loss of social experience. Interaction with others takes place in the dialysis center.

ADVANTAGES AND DISADVANTAGES OF TREATING DIABETICS

The dialysate contains glucose, which is used as an osmotic gradient for diffusion of urea and other solutes. The glucose is also absorbed by the peritoneum and can elevate serum sugar. Thus, dialysate is frequently given with insulin in diabetics. The advantage of insulin with the dialysate is having a basal steady state of insulin to keep glucose fluctuations at a minimum. The disadvantage of insulin is the risk of hypoglycemia. Furthermore, dialyzing diabetics via the peritoneum puts them at risk of absorbing too much dextrose and elevating serum glucose for prolonged periods.

PERITONEAL MEMBRANE

The peritoneal membrane is the term used to describe the lining of the abdominal cavity and pelvic walls including the diaphragm (parietal peritoneum) and the covering of the abdominal organs (visceral peritoneum). In males, it is completely sealed; in females, it opens into the Fallopian tubes and ovaries.

Exchange Process

The peritoneal membrane maintains contact with an abundance of blood vessels that supply the abdominal organs. In peritoneal dialysis, the dialysate is infused by means of a catheter, permitted to remain in the peritoneal cavity for a set amount of time, and then removed (effluent). This procedure is termed "an exchange." An osmotic gradient is created by using dextrose in the dialysate, which causes the shift of water into the peritoneal cavity. The surplus of water is removed when the effluent is drained. The process of diffusion causes electrolytes and uremic toxins to be removed from areas of higher concentration (bloodstream) to the area of lower concentration (peritoneal cavity). Low-molecular-weight solutes are "dragged" when solute removal is enhanced by use of a hypertonic dialysate, which increases ultrafiltration (UF) by means of convective transport.

Contraindications to Peritoneal Dialysis

There are many reasons to not initiate peritoneal dialysis in patients. Foremost, they need the support structure at home. Second, they must be open and willing to learn a new method of caring for themselves including troubleshooting (signs of infection, etc.). They must also have the manual dexterity and vision to carry out the requirements of peritoneal dialysis. Finally, clinical contraindications include peritoneal adhesions or fibrosis, abdominal neoplasm, documented poor peritoneal equilibration test, current or recurrent peritonitis and communication between the peritoneal and thoracic cavities.

Continuous Ambulatory Peritoneal Dialysis

Continuous ambulatory peritoneal dialysis (CAPD) is a dialysis method where the patient performs approximately 4-6 exchanges throughout the day. The term ambulatory differentiates this type of dialysis from automated peritoneal dialysis (continuous dialysis at night). The exchanges are carried out as per the nephrologist's orders. The dialysate enters the peritoneal cavity and sits there to allow for diffusion. After a predetermined time, the fluid is drained. The main drawback to CAPD is that one must perform an exchange every 4-6 hours.

Automated Peritoneal Dialysis

Automated peritoneal dialysis occurs when a machine automatically performs the exchanges. The machine is preprogrammed to deliver a set amount of fluid with timed frequencies. The dialysate used is prescribed by the nephrologist. The machine also warms the dialysate prior to infusion. The advantage to automated peritoneal dialysis is that it can be done at night without interfering with the patient's daily activities. Finally, a daytime dwelling dialysate can be left over to help clear larger molecules. The patient does not perform an exchange during the day but rather carries the excess dialysate fluid with them.

There are four types of automated peritoneal dialysis:

- Continuous cycling peritoneal dialysis—Three to five nightly exchanges with a daytime infusion to aid in molecular clearance.
- Nocturnal intermittent peritoneal dialysis—Three to five nightly exchanges with no daytime infusion. This is prescribed in patients who hyperabsorb the dextrose solution, suffer from congestive heart failure or have hernias and chronic low back pain.
- Intermittent peritoneal dialysis—Exchanges are performed three to five times per week. There is no left over dialysate in the peritoneum between exchanges. This is a more cost-effective method to dialysis and is also used in patients with residual renal function.
- Tidal peritoneal dialysis—Dialysate is initially infused into the peritoneum. After a predetermined time in the peritoneal cavity most of the dialysate is drained leaving some fluid behind. The fluid acts to increase clearance. When the next exchange occurs, a new dialysate is introduced (tidal dialysis). The cycle then repeats.

PERITONEAL DIALYSATE SOLUTIONS

The dialysate used contains dextrose (glucose) to facilitate the osmotic gradient necessary for dialysis. The dialysate also contains sodium, chloride, calcium, magnesium and lactate to approximate the extracellular electrolyte concentrations. Only potassium is absent or in lower concentrations to facilitate total body K removal. The solutions come in different dextrose concentrations: 1.5%, 2.5% and 4.25%. The increasing dextrose concentrations help facilitate a greater exchange. Finally, icodextrin is a new dialysate solution that does not contain dextrose. Instead, icodextrin employs a glucose polymer and aids in greater fluid removal.

COMMERCIALLY AVAILABLE SOLUTIONS

These solutions are created to be similar to extracellular fluid with the exception of potassium. Some of the commercially available peritoneal dialysis solutions are as follows:

- Dianeal PD-2
- Dianeal PD-1
- Dianeal Low Ca
- Icodextrin (Extraneal) does not contain dextrose, uses a starch derived osmotic agent
- Delflex

Potassium is not used in these dialysate solutions because many patients are hyperkalemic. Potassium may be added to the solution (2-4 mEq/L) if needed or an oral supplement may be prescribed. The more hypertonic the dialysate solution is, the greater the ultrafiltration that occurs. Dextrose is the ingredient that provides the osmotic gradient between plasma and dialysate facilitating the fluid and solute removal.

ICODEXTRIN

Icodextrin (Extraneal) is a dialysis solution that does not contain dextrose. Instead, it uses a starch based osmotic agent made from glucose polymers. This starch based solution allows for enhanced fluid removal from the blood during peritoneal dialysis, increases small solute clearance, and lowers the incidence of net negative ultrafiltration. Icodextrin is prescribed for use once in a 24-hour period via a long dwelling exchange lasting 8-16 hours. This product is contraindicated for those individuals with cornstarch allergies and those with glycogen storage diseases. Skin rash is the most commonly seen adverse effect with sterile peritonitis, hypertension, influenza-like symptoms, headache, and abdominal pain experienced by some patients.

PERITONEAL DIALYSIS CATHETER

A surgeon usually inserts a peritoneal dialysis catheter during a laparoscopy or laparotomy procedure. The usual exit site of is in midquadrant avoiding scars, skinfolds, or beltline. Catheters are either straight or coiled and have one or two cuffs. The coiled catheters are frequently preferred due to their minimal migration from the original insertion location and their lack of outflow problems. Coiled catheters also seem to cause less discomfort for the patient due to the configuration that keeps the tip of the catheter away from the peritoneal membrane. The cuffs, which are made of Dacron polyester or velour, allow ingrowth of tissue which stabilizes the catheter. In double cuffed catheters, the internal cuff is located in the rectus muscle with the external cuff placed in the subcutaneous tissue.

The four types of PD catheters used for long-term placement in the peritoneum include the following:

- Straight Tenckhoff catheter
- Curled Tenckhoff catheter
- Toronto western catheter
- Swan-neck (Missouri) catheter

Catheter "break-in" refers to the amount of time from when the chronic catheter is placed in the peritoneum until tissue ingrowth and healing have occurred. The goals during this "break-in" period of about six weeks are to promote healing and prevent complications such as dialysate leaks, infections or catheter obstruction. Full-volume dialysis should be avoided for a minimum of 10-14 days to allow healing to occur.

Factors That Influence Ultrafiltration and Solute Clearance

The following factors are implicated in clearance and ultrafiltration:

- Permeability of the peritoneal membrane (more permeable = better clearance)
- Volume of the exchange (higher volume = greater clearance)
- Dialysate glucose concentration (higher concentration = better clearance and fluid removal)
- Dwell time (longer times allow for more diffusion)
- Molecular size (small molecules are cleared more efficiently)

Other Forms of at Home Dialysis

The other main form of at home dialysis is home hemodialysis. This is rarely used today but was popular in the early 1970s. It is hemodialysis carried out by the patient at home. Problems with home hemodialysis include gaining access, sterile environment and having adequate support. The dialysis at home is usually a slow dialysis or a form of CRRT. This helps decrease the incidence of hypotension and ensures a more adequate dialysis.

Peritoneal Dialysis Complications

The most common complications include:

- Peritonitis
- Exit site infection
- Fibrin formation
- Tunnel infection
- Hemoperitoneum (blood in peritoneum)
- Inflow/outflow obstruction
- Pneumoperitoneum (air in peritoneum)
- Dialysate leak
- Hernia
- Pain on inflow

Exit Site Infections

Exit site infections occur when the skin flora (staph and strep) infect the exit site of the catheter. Signs of exit site infections include purulent drainage, skin induration and erythema along with abdominal pain. Exit site infections increase the risk of bacteria migrating into the peritoneum causing peritonitis. Treatment includes intraperitoneal along with systemic oral or intravenous antibiotics. Local care should also be increased with dressing changes occurring more frequently. Catheter removal may be necessary.

Peritonitis

Peritonitis is the most common complication of peritoneal dialysis. The indwelling catheter along with any exchanges increases the risk of introducing bacteria. Patients with peritonitis will present with abdominal pain, fever and nausea/vomiting. Laboratory studies will reveal elevated peritoneal white blood cell counts. Treatment includes intraperitoneal antibiotics to cover both gram-positive and gram-negative organisms.

Y-System

The Y-system is a set of connecting tubes and double bags, one of dialysate and the other empty. A stem connects to the peripheral dialysis catheter and transfer set with the afferent limb connected to the PD dialysate solution bag and the efferent limb attached to the empty drainage bag. There are clamps on both lines (limbs) to control the rate and direction of fluid flow allowing drainage or infusion. Priming the main stem with PD solution and allowing this solution to drain into the drainage bag instead of into the peritoneum has dramatically decreased the incidence of peritonitis.

Tunnel Infections

Pathophysiology and treatment of tunnel infections is explained below:

- Tunnel infections must be differentiated from exit site infections.
- Tunnel infections are subcutaneous and not readily visible.
- Tunnel infections are also not intraperitoneal and should not be confused with peritonitis.
- Signs of tunnel infections include erythema with underlying inflammation and swelling of the cuff.
- Treatment includes intravenous and intraperitoneal antibiotics.
- Tunnel infections also increase the risk of peritonitis.

Fibrin Formation

Fibrin formation occurs following peritonitis or a local inflammation from a previous infection. Fibrin clots or strands form during inflammatory processes and occur because of decreased clot degradation during the process. It is diagnosed when fibrin strands (white strands) are seen in the effluent. Treatment includes heparin being added to the dialysate.

Inflow/Outflow Obstructions

Inflow/outflow obstructions occur when fibrin clots form or catheter positioning changes. It is diagnosed when dialysate will neither enter nor exit the catheter. Treatment is usually with heparin flushes to break up the clots. If that does not work then plain films are taken and the catheter repositioned. Finally, the catheter may need to be replaced.

Hemoperitoneum

Hemoperitoneum means blood in the peritoneal cavity. The most common causes include retrograde menstruation, trauma with introducing the dialysis catheter, ruptured ovarian cysts and peritonitis. It is diagnosed when blood tinged or bright red blood is seen in the effluent. Hemoperitoneum is usually self-limiting but treatment includes frequent flushes with saline to prevent clot formation.

Dialysate Leak

A dialysate leak occurs when there is room around the catheter site or in the subcutaneous tissue for the dialysate to enter. Patients with a dialysate leak will often have increased abdominal pressure with clear fluid draining around the exit site or edema. It is diagnosed with a dextrostick and treated with cessation of peritoneal dialysis until the exit site heals or is resutured. Dialysate volume can also be decreased with each exchange to facilitate less fluid loss.

Pneumoperitoneum

Pneumoperitoneum means air in the peritoneal cavity. Each exchange will introduce some air into the peritoneal cavity. However, excess air can cause bowel obstruction and peritonitis. Pneumoperitoneum is diagnosed with excess bloating and shoulder pain. Plain abdominal films will confirm the diagnosis. Treatment involves draining the patient in Trendelenburg or knee-chest position. Moreover, looking for air leaks in the catheter is also important to rule loose connections.

Pain on Inflow

When dialysate is infused into the peritoneal cavity it can be painful. This is secondary to catheter migration near the peritoneal wall, acidic dialysate or rapid infusion. Treatment includes slower infusion rates, application of local anesthetics, and addition of bicarbonate or catheter change.

Hernias

Hernias occur when the dialysate fluid is introduced into the peritoneal cavity. The fluid-filled cavity will expand and any weakness in the abdominal wall musculature will be exploited by bowel. Ventral hernias are common. Most often surgery is not required for treatment as long as the hernia is readily reducible. However, surgery is the only definitive treatment.

Inflow and Outflow Problems

Peritoneal dialysis patients may experience inflow or outflow problems and may inadvertently get air in the abdomen. The catheter may become obstructed due to fibrin, blood, or omentum occluding the opening. Inflow and outflow problems may also be caused by the catheter's position, due to its migration out of the pelvis. Loculation caused by adhesions or constipation may also be considered as possible causes of obstruction of flow. Treatment options include the following:

- Relieving constipation
- X-ray for internal catheter kink
- Inspect catheter for external kinks
- Irrigate catheter with heparinized saline or a thrombolytic
- Reposition or replace catheter
- Peritoneogram with contrast medium to identify loculation

Air may enter the abdomen via loose connections or air in the system. The patient may complain of shoulder pain and peritoneal eosinophilia may be seen. Intervention includes draining the patient of the effluent and placing the patient in the knee-chest or Trendelenburg position. The air will be absorbed over time. Tighten all connections and inspect lines for presence of air.

Negatives Associated with PD

Some of the negatives associated with peritoneal dialysis (PD) include protein malnutrition and inadequate dialysis. The protein malnutrition results from the loss of amino acids and protein in the dialysate. The appetite is decreased due to the glucose load absorbed from the dialysis. This frequently results in hypertriglyceridemia, which causes weight gain from the caloric increase. Once residual renal function ceases, many patients are inadequately dialyzed using peritoneal dialysis. This results in the ESRD patient changing modes of dialysis from PD to HD in order to achieve optimal dialysis results.

Peritoneal Dialysis in Children

In children, peritoneal dialysis is the most commonly used method of chronic dialysis therapy. Most children use a cycling machine for overnight ADP. Complications of PD in children include the following:

- Catheter obstruction by omentum - usually prevented surgically by removing or trimming the omentum
- Inguinal and umbilical hernias - surgeon should review treatment
- Leakage around the catheter or exit site - usually indicates that the catheter has been used before the PD tract had sufficiently healed
- Peritonitis - prevention using excellent aseptic technique, comprehensive training for all caregivers, and closed-line delivery systems

- Growth problems due to reduced appetite with increased catabolic demands - monitoring and improving nutrition, correcting acidosis, and assessing bone disease and growth, using human growth hormone if indicated
- Hypertension is seen less frequently in children than in adults, but when severe, may require a prophylactic nephrectomy.

Interventions

ACCESSING THE PERITONEUM FOR PERITONEAL DIALYSIS

Peritoneal dialysis is done via a catheter, which is inserted near the umbilicus. This is a bedside procedure and there are various catheters. Catheters are inserted into the peritoneal cavity with tunneled cuffs to provide an adequate seal in the subcutaneous tissue. The tunneled cuffs also provide a barrier for invading infections. Catheters must remain in place for 10-14 days before being used. This allows for granulation and healing.

PERITONEAL EQUILIBRATION TEST

The peritoneal equilibration test is used to determine peritoneal membrane permeability. First, the patient's peritoneum is infused with 2.5% dialysate. Then dialysate samples of urea, glucose and creatinine are taken at 0, 2, 4 and 12 hours. The serum is also sampled for urea and glucose at 2 hours. The ratio of dialysate to peritoneal creatinine concentration is plotted against a standard chart. The same applies for glucose concentrations at 2 and 4 hours over glucose at 0 hours. The ratios are plotted against established standards and the peritoneal dialysate is adjusted accordingly.

DETERMINING PERITONEAL DIALYSIS ADEQUACY

The peritoneal equilibration test allows nephrologists to adjust peritoneal dialysate regimens and give insight to permeability. It does not, however, yield adequacy. Adequacy in dialysis is determined by the formula Kt/V. Kt/V is obtained by a 24-hour urine collection along with effluent (dialysis clearance). The current targets for adequacy as defined by the National Kidney Foundation are: continuous ambulatory peritoneal dialysis - Kt/V >2.0, continuous cycling peritoneal dialysis - Kt/V >2.1 and nocturnal intermittent peritoneal dialysis - Kt/V >2.2.

MEDICATIONS ADMINISTERED WITH PERITONEAL DIALYSIS

Dialysate is the fluid administered into the abdominal cavity to perform peritoneal dialysis. This is available in 1.5%, 2.5%, and 4.25 percent dextrose concentration. The higher the concentration of dextrose, the more fluid and waste will move into the abdominal cavity. Some of the regular medications that are taken on a daily basis by patients with peritoneal dialysis may include ACE inhibitors and diuretics. ACE inhibitors are used to treat hypertension and help to protect kidney function. Diuretics help the body to eliminate excess fluid and sodium. Peritoneal dialysis patients may also be taking vitamin D and phosphorous for bone strength. Vitamin D is produced by the kidneys, so patients on dialysis may not be producing the amount required to maintain bone strength. Iron may also be necessary if the patient is anemic. A hormone that is produced in the kidneys that stimulates red blood cell production, erythropoietin, may also need to be given for anemia. With kidney failure, it is very important that patients are educated on not taking any medications that have not been prescribed by their physician.

ALTERNATIVES TO ADMINISTERING ERYTHROPOIETIN IN PATIENTS ON PERITONEAL DIALYSIS

In patients on peritoneal dialysis, another method of administering erythropoietin is via the peritoneum. This is reserved for patients who do not tolerate the intravenous or subcutaneous route of administration. The peritoneum must be dry or with minimal dialysate. Moreover, the injection dose is usually increased by about 50% in those patients so as to achieve adequate levels of erythropoietin. The major drawback with giving intraperitoneal erythropoietin is lower absorption and the possibility of peritonitis. Anytime the peritoneal cavity is invaded, the prospect of bacterial or other form of peritonitis is increased substantially.

Limitations of Intraperitoneal Erythropoietin Injections

Intraperitoneal injections of erythropoietin require higher dosing than subcutaneous injections. The requirement is usually about 50 percent more and is necessary to ensure an adequate level of erythropoietin enters the system. Peritoneal injections of erythropoietin are also limited by decreased absorption by the peritoneal membrane and by the amount of fluid in the peritoneal cavity. Fluid in the peritoneal cavity acts to dilute the erythropoietin and will decrease its absorption. Therefore, it is always recommended that patients getting intraperitoneal erythropoietin should have a "dry" peritoneum or less than 50 ml of dialysate. Excess dialysate fluid will hinder proper absorption and decrease erythropoietin's efficacy.

Patient Education Before Peritoneal Dialysis

Once a decision has been made that peritoneal dialysis is right for the patient, a catheter is placed through the abdominal wall. The patient will need to be educated on caring for the catheter and cleaning around the catheter site to decrease the risk of infection. There is a risk of developing a hernia at the catheter site if there is straining to move the bowels, so they need to receive education on constipation prevention. Once the catheter site has healed, after about 2 weeks, education begins on how to perform peritoneal dialysis at home. The solution used, the dwell time (how long the fluid remains in the abdomen), and how to drain the fluid will need to be taught based on the type of dialysate used. The patient also needs to be educated on when to contact their healthcare provider with any problems. The development of abdominal pain, redness or swelling at the catheter site, cloudy dialysate fluid, or fever may indicate peritonitis, which needs to be treated urgently.

Home Peritoneal Dialysis

Outpatient training a patient for home peritoneal dialysis should be done once the patient has recovered from the catheter insertion surgery, which usually takes at least 2 weeks. An additional person who would be available to assist the patient at home, if needed, should also attend these sessions. The content must be customized to the patient's education level and learning abilities and should include the following:

- Basics of normal kidney function
- Effects of renal failure
- Mechanics of peritoneal dialysis
- Importance of aseptic technique
- Maintenance and care of catheter and exit site
- Record-keeping: body weight, blood pressure, treatments performed
- CAPD exchange procedures
- Use of a cycler if on APD
- Choice of dialysate solutions
- Recognition of signs and symptoms of infections
- Peritonitis and treatments
- Medications
- Ordering of supplies
- Dietary counseling
- Management of complications

Psychosocial Considerations When Considering Peritoneal Dialysis at Home

Some of the psychosocial issues to be considered when making the decision to use peritoneal dialysis at home are as follows:

- Patient's ability and motivation for self-care
- Employment or school requirements, scheduling conflicts
- Educational background
- Health beliefs
- Family and community support system
- Patient's state of mind, comprehension
- History of compliance with medical treatment
- Travel distance from dialysis facility
- Physical characteristics of home, availability of water source, electricity, phone, storage room for supplies, cleanliness
- Availability of additional caregiver, such as spouse, relative, friend

PD Quality Assurance Indicators

The goal of quality assurance should be continuous improvement. The Joint Commission on the Accreditation of Healthcare Organizations (JCAHO) and the Centers for Medicare and Medicaid (CMS) issue mandates that are implemented on a regional level by the ESRD networks to improve the care of the PD patient. Some quality assurance indicators are as follows:

- Incidence of treatment-related infections, such as peritonitis and exit site/tunnel infections
- Incidence of catheter complications, pericatheter leaks, migration, obstruction requiring replacement, and holes or cracks in catheters
- Patient morbidity, number of hospitalization days per year and cause of hospitalizations, and mortality
- Attainment of adequacy goals
- Constant review and revision of policies and procedures to improve quality of patient care

Transplant and Acute Therapies

Patients Not Considered Candidates for Renal Transplantation Surgery

Patients who cannot currently be considered for renal transplantation include the following:

- Those with active infections
- Patients with ongoing malignancies
- Patients who are current substance abusers
- Patients who are unable to adhere to medication schedules

Patients who may be considered, but whose transplantations are relatively contraindicated, include the following:

- Patients who are very young or over 65
- Patients with severe disease processes
- Patients with no family or other support mechanisms
- Patients with severe mental or psychological issues

HIV patients were not considered as candidates for renal transplantation surgery in the past because of the effect of the immunosuppressant drugs on the HIV infection. There currently is no policy that states patients who are HIV+ cannot receive transplants. Studies are being conducted at the University of Pittsburgh transplant center to determine the safety of liver and kidney transplants in the HIV+ patient.

Kidney Donation

The two sources for kidneys used in transplantation are living donors and deceased donors. There are only two requirements for a living donor to be considered as the source of a kidney. The donor must give voluntary informed consent and must be completely healthy. In order for a deceased person to be used as a kidney donor, the following requirements must be met:

- The patient must have had irreversible brain damage.
- Consent must have been given by the next of kin.
- The body must have been kept functioning by artificial ventilation and medications.
- The kidney must be recovered by organ recovery team.
- The kidney must go to a regional tissue and organ bank as per national guidelines to be distributed to a proper recipient.
- No expense is incurred by the donor family.

Immunological Basis of Organ Transplantation

The immune system guards the body against attacks from foreign invaders by identifying and destroying them. Anything that produces the 'identify and destroy' response by the immune system is termed an "antigen." Transplant researchers have identified two main antigen systems: blood groups (ABO), and human leukocyte antigen (HLA). The blood groups (ABO) are the first consideration when determining organ compatibility with the recipient with potential recipients divided by blood type. Rh (rhesus) factor does not affect solid organ transplantation. The HLA system comes from genes found in six locations on chromosomes. When tissue is introduced with unrecognized HLA genes, the rejection process begins. The most important components of the immune system are T-cells, which distinguish the tissue as foreign and start the rejection process, and B-cell lymphocytes, which recognize the foreign antigen and produce antibodies to destroy it.

Advantages and Disadvantages to Kidney Transplants

The major advantage to a kidney transplant is the increase in quality of life. Patients no longer have to attend thrice weekly hemodialysis or perform daily peritoneal exchanges at home. The lack of dependence on dialysis allows patients more independence and a greater sense of well-being. Transplant recipients also have a longer survival rate in contrast to dialysis patients. The disadvantage to transplantation is the lifelong dependence on immunosuppressive agents. Immunosuppression leaves patients susceptible to opportunistic infections including candida and possibly cancer. Moreover, the regimen of immunosuppressive agents can be both costly and complicated. Adverse effects from medications are quite common.

Immunologic Response to Transplanted Kidney

The transplanted kidney is a foreign body. The body's immune system recognizes antigens on the surface of the kidney as foreign. The immune system will defend itself by attacking the invading tissue. It specifically recognizes the human leukocyte antigen (HLA) and the ABO blood type as foreign. Thus, prior to transplantation a donor's blood type as well as HLA must match the recipient. Yet, even with matching antigens the immune system will react to the new kidney as a foreign invader. The role of immunosuppressants is to curtail the immune system's response. By suppressing the immunologic reaction, transplant nephrologists hope to preserve the new kidney's structure and function.

Contraindications to Receiving Kidney Transplant

The contraindications include:

- Infection
- Cancer
- Substance abuse (alcohol or drugs)
- Noncompliance
- Severe comorbidities

Panel Reactive Antibody

Panel reactive antibody (PRA) is the process of taking the recipient's blood and mixing it with random donors' lymph cells. The patient's serum will cross react with some donors while not reacting with others. The percent reaction defines the PRA level. The higher the percentage of reactivity, the less compatible a recipient will be to a donor. Therefore, if a patient has a high PRA level and they are matched with someone, they are given precedence. Patients with lower PRA scores will be more forgiving in accepting a larger range of potential kidneys.

Crossmatching

Crossmatching is the process of mixing recipient's blood with the donor's lymph cells to check for cross reactivity. First, samples from a recipient's blood are taken. Second, lymph cells are taken from the donor. The samples are then mixed. If the recipient's blood reacts to the lymph cells (attacks them), then that patient cannot receive the kidney. Although the recipient may not have been exposed to the donor's cells before, immune systems have a large range of antigen recognition. The immune system can recognize an antigen it has never seen before and attack it. This phenomenon occurs if that antigen is similar in structure to another antigen that the patient was previously exposed to.

Rejection

There are three general types of rejection:

- Hyperacute—Humoral based rejection. Preformed antibodies immediately attack the transplanted kidney within minutes. This is catastrophic and the transplant must be removed before it becomes infected. This is usually prevented with proper cross matching.
- Acute rejection—Cellular based rejection. T cells recognize the foreign kidney and start mounting an immune response. This rejection takes place within the first few months after transplantation.
- Chronic rejection—Humoral based rejection. This happens in all transplanted organs with time. The body forms antibodies against the transplant and slowly eats away at it. This is defined by a slow decline in kidney function with fibrosis noted in a biopsy.

Cellular and Humoral Rejection

There are two types of rejection: cellular and humoral.

- Cellular refers to T lymphocytes directly attacking the transplanted kidney. This is known as cell-to-cell combat.
- Humoral refers to antibodies attacking the transplanted kidney. The antibodies are released from B cells and like missiles attack the transplant. Immunosuppressive medicines target the actions of both T and B lymphocytes to limit the number and efficacy of attacks launched.

Diagnosis and Treatment

Rejection is commonly picked up by rising creatinine and oliguria. However, care must be taken to rule out other insults to the transplanted kidney including: medication induced, prerenal azotemia, obstruction, etc.

- Hyperacute rejection—Diagnosed immediately. The kidney quickly becomes necrotic with symptoms of a rapidly rising creatinine, fever, oliguria and pain. Treatment is to remove the kidney.
- Acute rejection—Diagnosed with oliguria, fever and tenderness over the transplant sight. This is the most common rejection and immunosuppressive agents are largely targeting this type of rejection. If the addition of steroids along with other immunosuppressive agents does not resolve the issue, the transplant may need to be removed.
- Chronic rejection—Diagnosed with a slowly rising creatinine. It is usually a diagnosis of exclusion and a biopsy is necessary. Only mycophenolate mofetil has been shown to lower chronic rejection rates.

Surgical Procedure Involved with Kidney Transplants

The transplanted kidney is placed in the iliac fossa. The iliac fossa is chosen to facilitate ease of placing the transplanted kidney as well as easier access in case it should be removed. Moreover, the iliac fossa is near the internal iliac artery and vein as well as the bladder to aid in the anastomosis of vessels and ureter. The transplanted renal artery and vein are anastomosed with their respective internal iliac artery and vein. The transplanted ureter is attached to the bladder. The procedure usually lasts from 2-4 hours and the entire hospital course is approximately 3-5 days.

Pre-Transplant Work up for Patients

Patients who are eligible for transplants should be referred to transplant centers. Transplant centers are equipped with multidisciplinary teams consisting of surgeons, transplant nephrologists, social workers, and nurse coordinators. They assist the patient and their family through the process. Preoperative workup includes the following:

- Complete cardiopulmonary assessment to ensure optimal or near optimal heart and lung function
- Signs of infection anywhere in the body
- Age-related cancer screening
- Psychological evaluation to screen for depression/anxiety as well as substance abuse

Dialysis After Kidney Transplant

A transplanted kidney is often slow to respond to its new environment. It may take days to produce adequate urine. In fact, there is no guarantee that a transplanted kidney will ever respond but the benefits far outweigh that risk. While the transplanted kidney is responding dialysis may be necessary. Dialysis in the post-operative patient must be careful so as not to compromise the new kidney. Thus, no anticoagulation or hypotension during dialysis can be tolerated.

Precautions

The most important part of post transplant dialysis is to ensure the safety of the transplanted organs. Any insult to the fragile transplanted kidney could place the whole process in jeopardy. Therefore, no heparin should be used during dialysis. Anticoagulation could result in internal bleeding at the operative site. Blood pressure must also be defended. Any hypotensive episode during dialysis places the transplanted kidney at high risk of ischemia and necrosis. Finally, electrolyte imbalances must be resolved.

Advantage of Having Combined Kidney/Pancreas Transplant

Quite commonly patients' renal failure is secondary to diabetes. In particular, type I diabetes causes renal failure in young persons. Therefore, a combined kidney/pancreatic transplant can alleviate both the renal failure as well as the hyperglycemia. The surgery is more complicated and the transplanted pancreas has a higher rate of rejection than the kidney alone. Moreover, the immunosuppressive regimen is far more complicated for the combined transplant. Yet, the potential benefits are great, particularly in young persons.

Duties of Nephrology Nurse Caring for Transplantation Patient

The nephrology nurse who cares for the transplantation patient plays several important roles including the following:

- Education of the patient regarding transplantation
- Counseling the patient about transplantation
- Assisting patient with the pretransplant evaluation
- Providing dialysis treatments for those patients with transient loss of renal function due to acute tubular necrosis (ATN)
- Providing dialysis treatments for patients who have experienced permanent loss of a transplanted kidney
- Providing dialysis treatments for patients who are experiencing acute or chronic renal failure due to transplanted non-renal organs (heart or liver)

Immunosuppressant Medications

The most common immunosuppressant classes are the following:

- Steroids—Blocks interleukin – 1 (a cytokine involved in the inflammatory cascade)
- Calcineurin inhibitors—Includes cyclosporine and tacrolimus block T cells reactions by blocking the signal calcineurin

- Antimetabolites—Include azathioprine and mycophenolate mofetil--act by blocking B cells
- Antilymphocytes—Include ATGAM and OKT3--block the actions of lymphocytes by targeting specific antigens on the lymphocytes
- Monoclonal antibodies—Include basiliximab and daclizumab-- are antibodies made to stop the actions of interleukin 2 (cytokine) and its binding with lymphocytes

EARLY SIGNS AND SYMPTOMS OF REJECTION AND INFECTION FOR THE POST-TRANSPLANT PATIENT

It is important for the transplant patient to understand that up to 20% of patients will experience at least one episode of rejection. This does not mean, however, that they will lose their new kidney or that the kidney is not functioning the way it should. The patient should contact their transplant team if they experience a fever greater than 101 degrees, flu-like symptoms, decreased urine output, weight gain, or pain over the transplant site. Most often, blood work shows signs of rejection before the patient experiences many symptoms. Blood tests included complete blood counts, kidney function tests, electrolyte levels, and drug levels of the immunosuppressant medications. Regular kidney biopsies are also performed to test the kidney tissue itself for any markers that may reveal the early signs of rejection. There is extensive research being done to find more blood tests that check specific cell markers and other biomarkers that may indicate the kidney is showing signs of rejection. Other diagnostic tests that may be performed to visualize the mechanical function of the kidney include ultrasound, CT scan, or MRI.

ORGAN TRANSPLANT PROCESS

Once the decision has been made to undergo a kidney transplant, the patient will work with a Clinical Transplant Coordinator. This person will be involved in coordinating all of the testing that is necessary to find a matching kidney, along with educating family members on the risks of organ donation. A Donor Coordinator is responsible for procuring and transporting the organ once a match has been found. Once the patient undergoes the surgical procedure to receive the new kidney, they will be in the ICU. The patient may need to continue dialysis until urine output is normal and the new kidney is functioning correctly. Fluids may be limited initially until the kidney is fully functioning. Immunosuppressant medications will be started and closely monitored to ensure the correct dosage is being received. The patient will receive consultation with a dietitian for any dietary guidelines they may need to follow. Physical therapy will also work with the patient to help with building strength. After discharge, there will be follow up appointments with the transplant surgeon to ensure the patient is healing appropriately and to be monitored for any signs of organ rejection.

RISKS FOR INFECTION AND INFECTION CONTROL TECHNIQUES FOR POST-TRANSPLANT PATIENTS

Due to the immunosuppressant therapy the transplant patient must take, there is a greatly increased risk of infection. Pediatric patients tend to be at greater risk than adult patients. Bacterial infections are more common than viral infections, with UTIs and vascular access infections being most prevalent. Cytomegalovirus infections are the most common viral infection. Before the transplant surgery, the patient should receive any vaccines which they are lacking. If vaccines are required post-surgery, inactivated vaccines should be given only. The risk of developing an infection from an active vaccine is greater than the benefit from receiving it post-transplant. The patient will be placed on prophylactic antibiotics to prevent UTI for up to one year following surgery. They may also be placed on antiviral therapy to prevent viral infection, usually for three months. Antifungal therapy may also be given depending upon the patient. The patient should be educated on their increased risk for infection and instructed in the importance of good handwashing. They should try to avoid others who they know are actively sick with an infectious disease. During epidemic levels of flu or other community illnesses, they should avoid large crowds to decrease their exposure.

ACUTE RENAL FAILURE

Acute renal failure is defined as a 50% decrease in glomerular filtration rate (GFR). There are three broad categories where the causes of acute renal failure fall into:

- prerenal
- intrinsic
- postrenal

The pathophysiology of acute renal failure is poorly understood but particular attention must be given to those patients whom may require replacement therapy. Acute renal failure results in the buildup of nitrogenous waste, other toxins and metabolites (chiefly potassium, phosphorus, BUN, creatinine). The most concerning metabolite is potassium, which is a known cardiac toxin and can result in dangerous arrhythmias and death.

COMMON CAUSES IN CHILDREN

The causes of acute renal failure in children are not that dissimilar from those causes seen in adults. These include:

- Prerenal azotemia from dehydration
- Sepsis
- Blood loss
- Nephrotoxic drugs such as aminoglycosides, nonsteriodal anti-inflammatory drugs (NDAIDS) and analgesics

However, the most common cause of acute renal failure in North American children is hemolytic uric syndrome, which can be seen with E.coli infections.

INDICATIONS FOR ACUTE DIALYSIS

The most common conditions in adults, infants and children that require acute dialysis are as follows:

- Symptomatic uremia, despite BUN and creatinine levels
- Pulmonary edema (a life-threatening complication of ARF), fluid overload, or acute myocardial infarction
- Hyperkalemia, when rapid reduction of plasma potassium level is indicated
- Acidosis, added sodium from IV sodium bicarbonate treatment may increase the chance of fluid volume overload
- Neurologic symptoms, toxic effects of uremia including headache, insomnia, lethargy, confusion, convulsions, and coma
- Drug overdose or poisoning, water-soluble drugs with low molecular weight (including ethanol, methanol, lithium and salicylates)

Drugs with high molecular weight (such as vancomycin and amphotericin B) or those that are protein bound (such as digoxin and acetylsalicylic acid), and lipid soluble drugs (for example, glutethimide) are not removed by dialysis.

INDICATIONS FOR URGENT DIALYSIS

The following are indications for urgent dialysis:

- A—Acidosis
- E—Electrolyte imbalance (hyperkalemia is the most common)

- I—Ingestion of poisons or drugs
- O—Volume Overload
- U—Uremic pericarditis or other uremic symptoms

DIALYSIS MOST AFFECTIVE IN ACUTE RENAL FAILURE

Acute renal failure has a mortality rate of 40-50%. In order to prevent uremia due to the compromised kidney function, the patient will require renal replacement therapy, or dialysis. With acute renal failure, there are several choices for hemodialysis therapy. Intermittent hemodialysis, continuous renal replacement therapies, and hybrid therapies are available. With intermittent hemodialysis, dialysis is performed in scheduled, intermittent intervals. Continuous renal replacement therapy is used while the patient is inpatient in the ICU until the acute renal failure resolves and therapy is no longer needed. The hybrid therapies are categorized into sustained low-efficiency dialysis and extended-duration dialysis. The sustained low-efficiency dialysis provides continuous dialysis without the hemodynamic instability that can occur with continuous renal replacement therapy. Extended-duration dialysis is also a viable method of renal replacement therapy that helps to avoid the hemodynamic instability that can occur with continuous renal replacement therapy. Because of the avoidance of the hemodynamic instability that can occur with continuous dialysis, the hybrid therapies are preferred as a dialysis method in the acute renal failure patient.

PREVENTING ACUTE DECREASE IN GLOMERULAR FILTRATION RATES IN PATIENTS WITH CHRONIC KIDNEY DISEASE

The following is a list of interventions (as per KDOQI) which help **prevent** any acute insult to the kidneys and cause a decline in GFR:

- Volume depletion (can cause prerenal acute renal failure)
- Radiocontrast
- Antibiotics such as amphotericin and aminoglycosides
- Avoidance of non-steroidal anti-inflammatory drugs
- Avoidance of ace inhibitors and angiotensin receptor blockers (only if they acutely decrease the glomerular filtration rate; otherwise they are indicated for use in patients with chronic kidney disease)
- Preventing urinary tract obstructions
- Avoidance of certain chemotherapeutic agents such as tacrolimus and cyclosporine

MEDICATIONS IMPORTANT IN TREATMENT OF ACUTE RENAL FAILURE

In conjunction with dialysis, the following are medications that are important in the treatment of acute renal failure:

- Phosphate binders: With kidney failure, phosphates will accumulate in the body. Phosphate binders, such as calcium carbonate, will help to eliminate phosphates.
- Vitamin D: This is produced by the kidneys, so a supplemental form is necessary with kidney failure to ensure adequate bone strength.
- RBC Stimulating Agents: These replace the hormone erythropoietin, which is normally produced by the kidneys to stimulate red blood cell production.
- Iron: This is given if iron levels are low from the anemia that occurs with kidney failure.
- Stool softeners and/or laxatives: Constipation can occur due to decreased fluid intake.
- Vitamins: Vitamins B, C, and folic acid are removed during dialysis and supplements may be necessary to replace these.
- Antihypertensives: Especially ACE inhibitors, which are protective of the kidneys.

- Antibiotics: These may be necessary to treat infections at a peritoneal dialysis catheter site, such as with peritonitis.
- Heparin: This is frequently given to prevent fibrin threads from forming, which can block the dialysis catheter.
- Insulin: Diabetic patients who are undergoing peritoneal dialysis, may require adjustments in their insulin (or initiation of insulin if they have not used it before) due to the absorption of dextrose from the dialysate causing blood sugar levels to increase.

Patient Education Following Acute Renal Failure and Dialysis

The following are key elements in patient education that must be communicated to the patient following acute renal failure and dialysis:

- Following the physician's orders for any special diets or fluid restrictions. Keep a log of all foods and drinks consumed.
- Monitor urine output and record this at home.
- Weight yourself daily to evaluate for any fluid retention.
- Take your temperature every day and notify your physician's office if it should be above normal.
- Educate the patient on how to take their blood pressure at home. This should be monitored and recorded daily.
- Avoid friends or family members who are sick with an acute illness.
- Teach good handwashing techniques to avoid the spread of infection.
- Take medications exactly as prescribed.
- Keep any follow up appointments that have been scheduled with your physician.
- Contact the physician's office if you should develop symptoms of a UTI, fever >100 degrees, chills or sweats, gain or loss of more than 3 pounds in 24 hours, or swelling of the extremities.
- If the patient is discharged with a urinary catheter, they should monitor around the catheter insertion site for any redness or purulent drainage.
- Keep other medical conditions under adequate control, such as hypertension or diabetes, by following the medication instructions of your physician.

CDN Practice Test

Section Description: Parker Case Questions

James Parker is a 48-year-old patient who has been receiving hemodialysis treatments 3 times weekly for the past 6 months.

1. Mr. Parker routinely experiences hypotensive episodes near the end of a session with malaise, muscle cramps, and dizziness after dialysis. What is the most likely cause?
   a. The dry weight is set too low.
   b. The dry weight is set too high.
   c. The patient is having an allergic reaction to dialysate.
   d. The patient is exhibiting signs of hypokalemia.

2. Generally, the optimal dialysate flow rate for hemodialysis should be
   a. equal to the blood flow rate.
   b. 1.5 to 2 times the blood flow rate.
   c. 2 to 2.5 times the blood flow rate.
   d. 2.5 to 3 times the blood flow rate.

3. According to the KDOQI, the minimum target (as opposed to delivered) spKt/V dose for patients receiving hemodialysis 3 times weekly is
   a. 0.8.
   b. 1
   c. 1.2
   d. 1.4

4. According to KDOQI guidelines, the dialysis dose for patients on hemodialysis should be monitored at least
   a. 1 time weekly.
   b. every 2 weeks.
   c. 1 time monthly.
   d. every 2 months.

5. If Mr. Parker is receiving hemodialysis with a dialyzer with an ultrafiltration coefficient (K_{UF}) of 10 and a transmembrane pressure (TMP) of 100 mm Hg, how much fluid should the patient lose per hour of treatment?
   a. 100 mL.
   b. 500 mL.
   c. 1000 mL.
   d. 1500 mL.

6. If Mr. Parker has a dialyzer clearance rate of 250 mL/min with 4-hour treatment, the total volume of blood cleared is
   a. 6 L.
   b. 60 L.
   c. 6000 mL
   d. 600 L.

7. Mr. Parker must have a postdialysis BUN. When drawing a postdialysis blood sample for BUN, one method is to slow the blood flow rate to
    a. 200 mL/min for 30 seconds.
    b. 100 mL/min for 15 seconds.
    c. 100 mL/min for 3 minutes.
    d. 200 mL/min for 3 minutes.

8. Mr. Parker must also have a number of other routine blood tests, including serum ferritin. The target for serum ferritin for patients on hemodialysis is
    a. ≥100 ng/mL.
    b. ≤100 ng/mL.
    c. ≥200 ng/mL
    d. ≤200 ng/mL.

9. Because Mr. Parker is a patient on hemodialysis, he must have a monthly albumin level tested. The target value for a patient on hemodialysis is
    a. >2.5 g/dL.
    b. >3.5 g/dL.
    c. >4 g/dL.
    d. >5 g/dL.

Section Description: Bell Case Questions

> Mary Bell is a 56-year-old woman scheduled for a kidney transplant because of autosomal dominant polycystic kidney disease. For the previous 4 years, the patient has been treated with hemodialysis.

10. Ms. Bell's partner has volunteered to be a living donor. The first concern when evaluating the donor is
    a. general health.
    b. insurance coverage.
    c. age and sex.
    d. psychological status.

11. Which of the following information gleaned during a psychiatric consultation is most likely to be a contraindication for kidney transplant?
    a. History of depression.
    b. History of nonadherence to treatment regimen.
    c. History of substance abuse.
    d. History of unemployment.

12. Following kidney transplantation, IV fluids are administered for maintenance and replacement of lost fluids. How much insensible loss is anticipated per hour?
    a. 10 mL.
    b. 30 mL.
    c. 45 mL.
    d. 60 mL.

13. In the immediate postoperative period after kidney transplantation, the physician should be notified if urinary output is
    a. <50 mL for 1 hour.
    b. >500 mL for 1 hour.
    c. >150 mL/h for 4 hours
    d. <60 mL/h for 2 consecutive hours.

14. Ms. Bell exhibit signs of kidney rejection 6 hours after transplantation. Kidney rejection within hours of transplantation is classified as...
    a. accelerated.
    b. hyperacute.
    c. chronic.
    d. acute.

15. Ms. Bell receives immunosuppressive agents to reduce risk of rejection. Which of the following immunosuppressive agents utilized to prevent kidney rejection after transplantation is the most nephrotoxic?
    a. Cyclosporine.
    b. Azathioprine.
    c. Tacrolimus.
    d. Mycophenolate mofetil.

16. When Ms. Bell is discharged after kidney transplantation, the nurse should ensure the patient understands that the primary measures to determine the health of the kidney are
    a. serum creatinine and urinary output.
    b. BUN and urinary output.
    c. BUN and serum creatinine.
    d. urinary output and blood pressure.

Section Description: Woods Case Questions

Tamara Woods is a 61-year-old woman who is critically ill and has developed acute kidney injury (AKI).

17. The most common cause of acute kidney injury in the critically ill is
    a. older age.
    b. heart failure.
    c. pneumonia.
    d. sepsis.

18. Ms. Woods has increasing peripheral edema and pulmonary congestion with decreased urinary output. The medication of choice is likely
    a. thiazide diuretic.
    b. osmotic diuretic.
    c. loop diuretic.
    d. potassium-sparing diuretic.

19. Ms. Wood's ECG telemetry shows peaked T waves and widening of the QRS interval. These changes may be indicative of
    a. hyperkalemia.
    b. hypokalemia.
    c. hypernatremia.
    d. hyponatremia.

20. Ms. Woods becomes anuric despite treatment, and her potassium level rapidly increases from 4.5 to 6. The most likely temporary emergent treatment is
    a. loop diuretic.
    b. insulin and glucose.
    c. sodium polystyrene sulfonate.
    d. intravenous normal saline.

21. If Ms. Woods' serum creatinine increases from 0.75 to 1.5 mg/dL, what effect on the GFR does the nurse expect?
    a. Increase 50%.
    b. Decrease 50%.
    c. Increase 25%.
    d. Decrease 25%.

Section Description: Rule Case Questions

James Rule is a 70-year-old male patient who developed hemolytic uremic syndrome (HUS) as the result of an Escherichia coli (O157:H7) infection.

22. HUS is characterized by the triad of (1) acute renal failure, (2) microangiopathic hemolytic anemia, and (3)
    a. thrombocytosis.
    b. thrombocytopenia.
    c. leukocytosis.
    d. leukopenia.

23. Initial therapy for HUS usually includes
    a. broad-spectrum antibiotics.
    b. antidiarrheal agents.
    c. antiplatelet agents.
    d. intravenous fluids.

24. With HUS, the part of the kidney that is damaged is the
    a. glomeruli.
    b. loops of Henle.
    c. distal tubules.
    d. papillae.

Section Description: Kim Case Questions

May Kim, a 58-year-old patient with type 2 diabetes and end-stage kidney disease (ESKD), has been treated with continuous ambulatory peritoneal dialysis (CAPD) for 2 years. The patient has developed numerous very painful firm brown nodules on both lower legs with some of the nodules eroding and become necrotic. The skin color appears mottled, and the patient has decreased sensation.

25. The most likely cause of these symptoms is
   a. calcific uremic arteriolopathy (CUA).
   b. peripheral arterial disease (PAD).
   c. peripheral venous insufficiency.
   d. *Staphylococcus aureus* infection.

26. Based on these symptoms, the most likely intervention is
   a. corticosteroids.
   b. immunosuppressive agents.
   c. IV antibiotics.
   d. IV or IP sodium thiosulfate.

Section Description: Anders Case Questions

Marian Anders, a 72-year-old woman with type 2 diabetes mellitus, has chronic kidney disease.

27. A patient with diabetes mellitus and chronic kidney disease should generally have a target HbA_{1c} of
   a. <5%.
   b. <6%.
   c. <7%.
   d. <8%.

28. In a diabetic patient with chronic kidney disease, glycosuria
   a. is a good estimation of hyperglycemia.
   b. is unreliable as an estimation of hyperglycemia.
   c. may occur without hyperglycemia.
   d. is almost always absent.

29. As chronic kidney disease progresses, which endocrinologic change can result in higher risk of fractures?
   a. Hyperparathyroidism.
   b. Hypoparathyroidism.
   c. Hypothyroidism.
   d. Hyperthyroidism.

30. Mrs. Anders' hemoglobin is 11 g/d. According to KDIGO guidelines, treatment for chronic kidney disease with an erythropoiesis-stimulating agent should not be initiated until the hemoglobin level falls to
   a. <9 g/dL.
   b. <10 g/dL.
   c. <11 g/dL.
   d. <12 g/dL.

31. Ms. Anders must have dialysis or transplantation in order to survive when kidney function falls below
    a. 30% to 40%.
    b. 20% to 30%.
    c. 15% to 20%.
    d. 10% to 15%

32. Dialysis will likely begin when Ms. Anders has a GFR (MDRD equation) of
    a. <15 mL/min/1.732.
    b. <20 mL/min/1.732.
    c. <25 mL/min/1.732.
    d. <30 mL/min/1.732.

Section Description: Aiken Case Questions

Drake Aiken, an 18-year-old male patient with ESKD resulting from IgA nephropathy, is to begin using CAPD to control his condition.

33. When assisting a surgeon with stencil-based preoperative mapping for insertion of a peritoneal dialysis catheter, the nurse should initially position Mr. Aiken...
    a. in any convenient position.
    b. standing.
    c. sitting.
    d. supine.

34. Prior to surgical placement of a catheter for peritoneal dialysis, the recommended antibiotic prophylaxis is generally
    a. a cephalosporin (first generation).
    b. vancomycin.
    c. a sulfonamide.
    d. an aminoglycoside.

35. After a catheter is implanted, a culture of the catheter exit site is positive for *Staphylococcus aureus* but there is no erythema or purulent discharge. The most likely cause of the positive culture is
    a. peritonitis.
    b. lab error.
    c. colonization.
    d. specimen contamination.

36. Mr. Aiken receives instruction from the nurse about self-care and managing CAPD in the home environment. Which of the following is an acceptable method of warming dialysate for peritoneal dialysis in the home?
    a. Immerse in warm water.
    b. Apply a heating pad.
    c. Leave at room temperature for 3 hours.
    d. Hold under running warm water.

37. Once a dialysate bag is heated, the temperature can be assessed by
   a. holding the bag against the wrist.
   b. folding the bag over and enclosing an electronic thermometer.
   c. inserting a thermometer into the tubing.
   d. laying an electronic thermometer on top of the bag.

38. With CAPD, the number of exchanges that Mr. Aiken should expect to carry out in 24 hours is usually
   a. 2 to 3.
   b. 3 to 4.
   c. 4 to 5.
   d. 5 to 6.

39. With CAPD, the volume of dialysate retained in the peritoneal cavity at all times in adults, such as Mr. Aiken, is usually approximately
   a. ≤0.5 L.
   b. ≤1 L.
   c. ≤2 L.
   d. ≤3 L.

Section Description: Maddox Case Questions

Jane Maddox is a 52-year-old woman who has started on hemodialysis after both kidneys were removed because of bilateral renal cell carcinoma.

40. When teaching Ms. Maddox to manage fluid balance, the nurse advises the patient that a 1 kg (2.2 lb) increase in weight in 24 hours is approximately equivalent to fluid retention of
   a. 0.5 L.
   b. 1 L.
   c. 1.5 L.
   d. 2 L.

41. Ms. Maddox has been advised to avoid foods high in phosphorus. Foods that she should be advised to limit include
   a. dairy products.
   b. vegetables.
   c. fruits.
   d. grains.

42. Ms. Maddox has been prescribed sevelamer hydrochloride as a phosphate binder. The patient should be advised to take this medication
   a. 1 hour before meals.
   b. 2 hours after meals.
   c. first thing in the morning.
   d. with meals.

43. If Ms. Maddox usually drinks 2 cups of caffeinated coffee each morning and has headaches during hemodialysis, she should be advised to
    a. stop drinking coffee altogether.
    b. drink a cup of strong coffee with treatment.
    c. skip coffee the morning of the treatment.
    d. transition to decaffeinated beverages.

Section Description: Independent Questions, Group 1

44. A patient who cannot tolerate contrast for a CT is scheduled for an MRI to evaluate a mass on his kidney. The nurse notes that the patient seems very nervous and upset as the time for the MRI approaches. On questioning, the patient confesses to the nurse that, although he understands the need for the MRI, he is very claustrophobic and worried about the procedure. The best solution is to
    a. reassure the patient that the MRI procedure is benign.
    b. advise the patient to close his eyes and practice relaxation during the MRI.
    c. contact the physician and request an order for a sedative.
    d. cancel the MRI.

45. The first indication of renal cancer is often
    a. flank pain.
    b. painless hematuria.
    c. unexplained weakness.
    d. anemia.

46. For a patient with ESKD diagnosed with tuberculosis, which of the following antitubercular drugs can be administered at 100% of the normal dose?
    a. Ethambutol.
    b. Pyrazinamide.
    c. Isoniazid.
    d. Rifabutin.

47. According to the RIFLE criteria for acute kidney dysfunction, urinary output indicative of kidney failure is ...
    a. <0.5 mL/kg/h for 6 hours.
    b. <0.5 mL/kg/h for 12 hours.
    c. <0.3 mL/kg/h for 24 hours.
    d. anuria for 6 hours.

48. If a patient's cardiac output decreases, resulting in arterial hypoperfusion with reduced blood flow to the kidneys, the nurse expects lab results to show...
    a. increased BUN.
    b. decreased BUN.
    c. increased GFR.
    d. stable BUN and decreased GFR.

49. Which of the following is an example of an intrarenal cause of acute kidney injury (AKI)?
   a. Hemorrhage.
   b. Sepsis.
   c. Urethral obstruction.
   d. Tumor lysis syndrome.

50. Which of the following medications may result in tubular cell toxicity?
   a. Acetaminophen.
   b. Aminoglycosides.
   c. Diphenhydramine.
   d. Benzodiazepines.

51. Prior to a serum creatinine test, the patient should be advised to
   a. avoid excessive exercise.
   b. avoid food and fluids for 12 hours.
   c. drink 3 to 4 glasses of water.
   d. avoid fluids for 6 hours.

52. The primary preventive measure to avoid contrast-induced nephrotoxic injury for a patient who must receive IV radiopaque contrast material despite chronic kidney dysfunction is
   a. IV sodium bicarbonate.
   b. oral N-acetylcysteine.
   c. IV normal saline.
   d. IV fenoldopam.

53. Which of the following ethnic groups is most at risk for development of kidney failure?
   a. Caucasians.
   b. Hispanic Americans.
   c. Asians.
   d. African Americans.

54. Patients may be advised to fast for at least 4 hours prior to a CT of the kidney with IV iodinated contrast because
   a. fasting improves images.
   b. physician preference, fasting not necessary.
   c. patients may experience nausea and vomiting.
   d. some foods may interact with the contrast material.

55. Which of the following are the primary causes of nephrosclerosis?
   a. Hypertension and hepatitis B.
   b. Hypertension and diabetes.
   c. Hypertension and HIV.
   d. Hypertension and kidney trauma.

56. Shortly after emergency department admission for post-infectious acute glomerulonephritis, a patient develops altered mental status. The most likely cause of this complication is
    a. anemia.
    b. dehydration.
    c. hypertensive encephalopathy.
    d. hyponatremia.

57. Prerenal kidney failure may result from
    a. nephrotoxic agents.
    b. urinary tract obstruction.
    c. prolonged renal ischemia.
    d. volume depletion.

58. Which of the following laboratory findings is characteristic of acute prerenal kidney failure?
    a. Na <20 mEq/L.
    b. Na >20 mEq/L.
    c. Na <40 mEq/L.
    d. Na >40 mEq/L.

59. The obligatory urinary output that is needed to filter normal metabolic waste products and remove them from the body is about
    a. 300 mL.
    b. 500 mL.
    c. 700 mL.
    d. 800 mL.

60. Which of the following medications is nephrotoxic and should have baseline and follow-up BUN and serum creatinine monitored during administration?
    a. Metoprolol.
    b. Acetaminophen.
    c. Calcitriol.
    d. Vancomycin.

61. With kidney disease, decreased specific gravity may result from
    a. volume excess.
    b. glycosuria.
    c. volume deficit.
    d. proteinuria.

62. If a patient with kidney failure has an order for a sodium polystyrene sulfonate (Kayexalate) retention enema, the nurse expects that the patient is being treated for
    a. hypokalemia.
    b. hyperkalemia.
    c. hypophosphatemia.
    d. hyperphosphatemia.

63. A patient with acute kidney failure is stabilizing and seems alert and responsive, but the nurse notes that the patient needs to have explanations for treatments and procedures repeated many times. The most likely reason is
   a. anemia.
   b. encephalopathy.
   c. dementia.
   d. anxiety.

Section Description: Evans Case Questions

Sally Evans, a 48-year-old woman, has been using peritoneal dialysis for the past year. Swabs of her nares indicate that she is colonized with Staphylococcus aureus.

64. Ms. Evans notes the dialysis effluent is cloudy when it drains. For a patient undergoing peritoneal dialysis, when sending a sample of cloudy dialysate for culture and sensitivities, what is the minimal sample size?
   a. 5 mL.
   b. 10 mL.
   c. 20 mL.
   d. 30 mL.

65. Ms. Evans develops tenderness around the catheter site and purulent discharge. Which of the following additional signs/symptoms are included in the minimal diagnostic criteria for peritonitis?
   a. Fever and dialysate WBC of 50 cells/mm3 and 25 PMN leukocytes.
   b. Cloudy dialysate and dialysate WBC of 50 cells/mm3 and 25 PMN leukocytes.
   c. Abdominal pain and dialysate WBC of 50 cells/mm3 and 30 PMN leukocytes.
   d. Abdominal pain and dialysate WBC of >100 cells/mm3 and 50 PMN leukocytes.

66. Ms. Evans is diagnosed with peritonitis. When Ms. Evans is being treated for peritonitis, fibrinous clots are visible in the dialysis effluent. The treatment of choice is
   a. heparin.
   b. warfarin.
   c. dabigatran.
   d. apixaban.

Section Description: Elmers Case Questions

Mary Jane Elmers is a 28-year old patient on hemodialysis. She is 3 months pregnant.

67. Ms. Elmers should be advised to wash the access site before coming for treatment with
   a. isopropyl alcohol 70%.
   b. povidone iodine.
   c. chlorhexidine gluconate 2%.
   d. soap and water.

68. Ms. Elmers' blood pressure is 160/100 mm Hg when she is euvolemic. An acceptable medication to treat hypertension in a pregnant patient on hemodialysis is

   a. labetalol.
   b. atenolol.
   c. ACE inhibitors.
   d. Angiotensin receptor blockers (ARBs).

69. In order to increase the chance that Ms. Elmers will deliver a viable infant, ideally, she should be dialyzed

   a. on the same schedule as before pregnancy.
   b. 15 hours per week.
   c. <20 hours per week.
   d. >20 hours per week.

70. Ms. Elmers finds that sipping ginger ale during hemodialysis relieves her nausea. How should fluid consumed during hemodialysis be accounted for?

   a. The volume of ginger ale should be ignored.
   b. The total volume must be added to the total volume of fluid that must be removed.
   c. The total volume is accounted for in the next hemodialysis treatment.
   d. Half the volume should be added to the total fluid that must be removed.

71. Ms. Elmers is concerned about what prenatal vitamins to take. Which of the following vitamin supplements should be avoided in patients undergoing hemodialysis?

   a. Vitamin B6.
   b. Folic acid.
   c. Vitamin C.
   d. Vitamin A.

Case Description: Shaw Case Questions

   Stanley Shaw is a 64-year-old man who has been using automated peritoneal dialysis (APD) for the past 2 years.

72. For a patient such as Mr. Shaw, receiving APD with most dialysis occurring during the night, the best time to take a plasma sample to determine the urea level is

   a. at bedtime.
   b. on arising.
   c. noon.
   d. mid-afternoon.

73. With APD, icodextrin may be used rather than glucose solution for

   a. all short daytime dwells.
   b. 1 long day dwell.
   c. long nocturnal dwell.
   d. all dwells, day and night.

74. With APD, how many nighttime hours would Mr. Shaw spend cycling?
   a. 4 to 6.
   b. 6 to 8.
   c. 8 to 10.
   d. 10 to 12.

Section Description: Mayweather Case Questions

Dan Mayweather is a 48-year-old male patient who received peritoneal dialysis for 5 years but has recently changed to in-center hemodialysis. Mr. Mayweather is preparing to switch to home hemodialysis.

75. Mr. Mayweather has developed pain and stiffness in the joints. The most likely cause is
   a. osteoarthritis.
   b. rheumatoid arthritis.
   c. amyloidosis.
   d. gout.

76. Mr. Mayweather complains of severe itching during and after hemodialysis despite taking a phosphate binder. Which medication is commonly prescribed to help relieve the itching?
   a. Prednisone.
   b. Calcitriol.
   c. Diazepam.
   d. Diphenhydramine.

77. A primary advantage of home hemodialysis is
   a. more frequent treatments.
   b. lower risk of infection.
   c. lower cost.
   d. longer fistula survival.

78. The nurse is teaching Mr. Mayweather about aseptic techniques. If using a combination chlorhexidine gluconate and alcohol skin prep (such as ChloraPrep) before cannulation, how much skin contact time is required?
   a. 15 seconds.
   b. 30 seconds.
   c. 60 seconds.
   d. 3 minutes.

79. Mr. Mayweather has opted to have a buttonhole technique for hemodialysis. Which of the following is the most important factor for creation of a buttonhole technique for hemodialysis?
   a. The originator should document the exact site and angle of needle insertion.
   b. A team of at least 2 cannulators should alternate treatments until the tunnel is established.
   c. The patient should do all cannulations until the tunnel is established.
   d. The same cannulator should do treatments until the tunnel is established.

80. Mr. Mayweather has buttonhole tracks for access and is being taught to carry out treatments with the assistance of his wife. After the area is cleansed and prepped for treatment, what is the next step?
   a. Insert sharp needles into the tracks.
   b. Insert blunt needles into the tracks.
   c. Use a scab picker/aseptic tweezers to remove the scabs.
   d. Use the treatment needle to remove the scabs.

81. With buttonhole tracks, Mr. Mayweather should be taught to apply pressure as the needles are removed and then for
   a. 1 to 2 minutes.
   b. 5 to 10 minutes.
   c. 10 to 20 minutes.
   d. 20 to 30 minutes.

82. If Mr. Mayweather's buttonhole access frequently has long clots that are very difficult to remove, the most likely reason is
   a. subclinical infection.
   b. use of improper needle.
   c. failure to use 2-finger hold for needle removal.
   d. failure to adequately remove previous clot before cannulation.

83. With buttonhole access sites, what should Mr. Mayweather do to prevent "hubbing?"
   a. Leave 1/16th to 1/8th inch of the needle exposed.
   b. Insert the needle just to the hub.
   c. Use a sharp needle to remove scabs.
   d. Use a long catheter so the hub is not close to the site.

84. Mr. Mayweather complains that he frequently experiences muscle cramping during hemodialysis. The most common predisposing factor for muscle cramping during hemodialysis is
   a. electrolyte imbalance.
   b. low ultrafiltration rate.
   c. high sodium dialysis solution.
   d. hypotension.

85. The nurse is teaching Mr. Mayweather about complications that may arise during hemodialysis. Which of the following is an indication that there is clotting in the extracorporeal circuit?
   a. Very light bright blood.
   b. White streaks in the dialyzer.
   c. Foaming and clots in drip chamber.
   d. Teetering blood in the arterial line segment.

86. The nurse advises Mr. Mayweather that foam in the venous blood line of a dialyzer may indicate
   a. normal finding.
   b. sepsis.
   c. too rapid blood flow rate.
   d. air embolism.

87. When a patient is using home hemodialysis, the purpose of teaching the patient to "snap and tap" the tubing and filter is to
    a. remove air bubbles.
    b. straighten the tubing.
    c. prime the tubing with saline.
    d. improve patency.

Section Description: Jones Case Questions

Ben Jones, a 58-year-old patient with ESKD, has numerous complaints about his quality of life and is generally unhappy. Mr. Jones has had difficulties managing his treatment regimen.

88. Which of the following psychiatric disorders is most common in patients with ESKD?
    a. Anxiety.
    b. Dementia.
    c. Depression.
    d. Bipolar disorder.

89. Mr. Jones is screened with the Beck Depression Inventory and has a score of 20, suggesting
    a. no depression.
    b. mild depression.
    c. moderate depression.
    d. severe depression.

90. Mr. Jones participates in cognitive behavioral therapy to decrease depression, but his depression worsens, so the physician has prescribed an SSRI. For a patient with ESKD, the dosage of the SSRI should be
    a. Reduced by two-thirds.
    b. Increased by two-thirds.
    c. Reduced by one-third.
    d. Decreased by one-third.

91. Mr. Jones has not adhered to his diet plan, and the nurse is encouraging him to maintain a high-carbohydrate diet. The purpose of a high-carbohydrate diet for a patient with ESKD is to
    a. improve appetite.
    b. improve sense of well-being.
    c. spare protein for growth and healing.
    d. spare fat for growth and healing.

Section Description: Independent Questions, Group 2

92. Femoral catheters for vascular access for hemodialysis should be left in place for no longer than
    a. 2 days.
    b. 5 days.
    c. 2 weeks.
    d. 4 weeks.

93. If a patient develops an infection of a primary AV fistula and requires more than 6 weeks of antibiotic treatment, which of the following conditions should be suspected?
    a. Subacute endocarditis.
    b. Sepsis.
    c. Pericarditis.
    d. Encephalitis.

94. For short-term central venous catheters in adults, the CDC recommends that transparent dressings be changed at least every
    a. 24 hours.
    b. 2 days.
    c. 5 days.
    d. 7 days.

95. If a patient with acute tubular necrosis is receiving hemodialysis, which phase of the disease may be obscured?
    a. Oliguria/Anuria.
    b. Diuresis.
    c. Recovery.
    d. Onset.

96. For a hemodialysis cannulation with a blood flow rate of less than 300 mL/min, which of the following needle gauge sizes is usually recommended?
    a. 14.
    b. 15.
    c. 16.
    d. 17.

97. If a dialysis center is utilizing Continuous Quality Improvement (CQI) methods, the question that the nurse should continually ask is
    a. "How can I avoid errors?"
    b. "How can the center be more cost effective?"
    c. "How can the center do things better?"
    d. "What is the staff doing right?"

98. The first step in the CQI process is to
    a. identify the need for improvement.
    b. analyze the process.
    c. identify root causes.
    d. implement plan-do-check-act (PDCA).

99. Early symptoms of disequilibrium syndrome associated with long-term hemodialysis include
    a. seizures and coma.
    b. hypertension and tachycardia.
    c. headache, nausea, and vomiting.
    d. headache and respiratory distress.

100. An 80-year-old patient with ESKD is a candidate for hemodialysis, but the patient refuses treatment, stating that death is preferable to the loss of independence and continued illness. The nurse should
    a. suggest the patient see a psychiatrist.
    b. try to convince the patient of the benefits of hemodialysis.
    c. remind the patient that he will die soon without treatment.
    d. respect the patient's decision.

101. If a patient with diabetes mellitus at high risk for kidney disease shows negative for macroscopic protein with dipstick testing, the nurse expects the next step to be
    a. doing dipstick testing at all follow-up visits.
    b. assuming the patient is not at risk.
    c. testing for microalbuminuria.
    d. serum creatinine.

102. For which of the following sleep disorders should all hemodialysis patients be screened?
    a. Insomnia.
    b. Restless legs syndrome (RLS).
    c. Obstructive sleep apnea.
    d. Periodic limb movements in sleep (PLMS).

103. The most important factor in preventing exsanguination from dialysis line separation is
    a. functioning venous alarms.
    b. access site visibility.
    c. use of HemaClips.
    d. patient education.

104. If a sentinel event (such as death resulting from exsanguination) occurs, the initial response must include
    a. conducting a root cause analysis.
    b. firing the staff involved.
    c. determining who was to blame.
    d. consulting attorneys.

105. The pH of dialysate usually ranges from
    a. 6.5 to 6.8.
    b. 6.8 to 7.
    c. 7 to 7.4.
    d. 7.4 to 7.6.

106. A patient on hemodialysis has suffered a myocardial infarction (MI) and remains weak. She has not resumed any exercise because of fear of another MI. The patient may benefit the most from a referral to a
    a. psychiatrist.
    b. support group.
    c. physical therapist.
    d. cardiac rehabilitation program.

107. Which of the following agencies/organizations sets the minimally adequate target spKt/V as a clinical performance measure for all out-patient dialysis centers in the United States?

   a. FDA.
   b. OSHA.
   c. CDC.
   d. CMS.

108. The electronic event-reporting documentation form for the dialysis center is lengthy and time-consuming and not always applicable to the center, causing staff members to avoid making reports of near-misses despite guidelines that require them to do so. The best solution is to

   a. keep alternate records for near misses.
   b. assign a staff person to ensure all events are recorded.
   c. identify those elements of the form that require modification.
   d. complain to the administration that the form is too time-consuming.

109. A patient complains of pain and tightness in the chest with pain radiating to the jaw and down the left arm during hemodialysis. Before notifying the physician, the nurse's immediate intervention should be to

   a. slow the blood flow rate to 150 mL/min and decrease the ultrafiltration rate.
   b. increase the blood flow rate and the ultrafiltration rate by 20%.
   c. clamp all lines and stop dialysis.
   d. continue treatment without alteration.

110. The potassium level in dialysate is commonly

   a. 4 mM.
   b. 3 mM.
   c. 2 mM.
   d. 1 mM.

111. Because a new dialyzer is to be reused, it is preprocessed and tested to determine the baseline total cell volume (TCV) (or fiber bundle volume) value. To be used again, a subsequent TCV must be at least

   a. 60% of baseline.
   b. 70% of baseline.
   c. 80% of baseline.
   d. 90% of baseline.

112. A normal adult man makes about how much glomerular filtrate every 24 hours?

   a. 125 mL.
   b. 125 L.
   c. 180 mL.
   d. 180 L.

113. The 2 hormones secreted by the kidneys are erythropoietin and

   a. calcitriol.
   b. calcium.
   c. aldosterone.
   d. gastrin.

114. The number 1 cause of kidney failure in the United States is
   a. polycystic kidney disease.
   b. diabetes mellitus, type 1.
   c. diabetes mellitus, type 2.
   d. cardiovascular disease.

115. A dialysis center offers nighttime hemodialysis with 7- to 8-hour sessions 3 times weekly. Compared with the usual daytime schedule, the nighttime schedule
   a. results in more complications.
   b. results in better survival rates.
   c. results in more food and fluid restrictions.
   d. offers no advantage.

Section Description: Washington Case Questions

Jasper Washington is a 56-year-old man with type 2 diabetes mellitus. Mr. Washington is newly diagnosed with ESKD and in need of peritoneal dialysis.

116. Mr. Washington has little income, inadequate insurance, and little social support. The best initial referral is to
   a. Medicaid.
   b. home health agency.
   c. social worker.
   d. free clinic.

117. When instructing Mr. Washington in the use of a preattached double bag system for peritoneal dialysis, he should be advised to flush how much dialysate from the fill bag to the drainage bag before filling the peritoneal cavity?
   a. 25 mL.
   b. 50 mL.
   c. 75 mL.
   d. 100 mL.

118. When teaching Mr. Washington about dialysate, the nurse should understand that the primary advantage of a 2-compartment peritoneal dialysis solution bag is to
   a. allow delivery at normal pH.
   b. maintain pH at 5.5.
   c. decrease risk of infection.
   d. allow 2 different solutions to be instilled sequentially.

119. The nurse teaches Mr. Washington that the 3 transport processes that occur during the course of peritoneal dialysis are (1) diffusion, (2) ultrafiltration, and (3)
   a. radiation.
   b. transference.
   c. absorption.
   d. conduction.

Section Description: Garcia Case Questions

Jose Garcia is a 64-year-old man on hemodialysis because of kidney failure related to exposure to toxic chemicals in an industrial accident.

120. Mr. Garcia is receiving hemodialysis with 17-gauge needles, but his blood flow rate has increased to 450 mL/min. The patient suddenly complains of chest tightness, back pain, and dyspnea, and the nurse notes flushing and port-wine colored blood in the venous line. Which complication is most likely?

   a. Disequilibrium syndrome.
   b. Hemolysis.
   c. Air embolism.
   d. Cardiac tamponade.

121. Based on Mr. Garcia's symptoms (sudden onset of chest tightness, back pain, and dyspnea, reddening of skin color, and blood in the venous line appearing port-wine in color), the immediate action should be to

   a. slow the blood flow rate to <400 mL/min.
   b. administer normal saline.
   c. stop the blood pump and clamp the blood lines.
   d. monitor electrolytes.

122. For which electrolyte imbalance should Mr. Garcia be monitored?

   a. hyperkalemia.
   b. hypokalemia.
   c. hypophosphatemia.
   d. hyperphosphatemia.

123. According to KDOQI guidelines, Mr. Garcia should receive treatment with an active vitamin D sterol (such as calcitriol) when parathyroid hormone (PTH) levels are

   a. >150 pg/mL.
   b. >200 pg/mL.
   c. >300 pg/mL.
   d. >400 pg/mL.

124. Which of the following statements by Mr. Garcia most suggests that the patient may need a referral for psychological counseling?

   a. "I hate having to come for treatments 3 times a week."
   b. "It's hard for me to keep up at work."
   c. "Some days I wish I didn't even wake up."
   d. "Living with kidney failure is pretty miserable at times."

125. Mr. Garcia persists in smoking despite attempts to educate the patient about the risks of smoking. Mr. Garcia points out that his parents and family members smoke, and all are relatively healthy. The nurse should advise the patient that
   a. risks of smoking are essentially the same for dialysis patients as for people without kidney disease.
   b. nicotine levels after smoking are higher in dialysis patients than in people without kidney diseases.
   c. the patient is at much greater risk from smoking than his family members.
   d. the patient should not compare himself with healthy family members.

Section Description: Independent Questions, Group 3

126. The amount of dialysis that a hemodialysis patient is prescribed is based on the removal of
   a. urea.
   b. creatinine.
   c. potassium.
   d. albumin.

127. The use of topical anesthetics, such as EMLA, to reduce discomfort during cannulation is contraindicated with
   a. AV fistulas.
   b. AV grafts.
   c. all hemodialysis patients.
   d. buttonhole sites.

128. If a patient tests positive for the hepatitis B core antibody (HBcAb) test, this means that the patient
   a. has been exposed to hepatitis B.
   b. is immune to hepatitis B.
   c. is infected with hepatitis B.
   d. is receiving treatment for hepatitis B.

129. As chronic kidney disease progresses from stage 2 to stage 3, the focus of clinical intervention moves toward
   a. reducing risk and slowing progression.
   b. monitoring progression.
   c. preparing for dialysis.
   d. evaluating and treating complications.

130. Healthcare personnel caring for patients undergoing kidney transplantation should receive which of the following immunizations?
   a. Influenza (annual).
   b. Herpes zoster.
   c. Hepatitis C.
   d. DTaP.

131. If a patient with a donor kidney develops sudden onset of hypertension 2 years after transplantation, the most likely cause is
   a. vascular thrombosis.
   b. ureteral obstruction.
   c. graft rejection.
   d. arterial stenosis.

132. Following kidney transplantation, a patient develops a large lymphocele between the bladder and the transplanted kidney. The treatment of choice is usually
   a. internal drainage into abdomen.
   b. sclerotherapy.
   c. instillation of fibrin glue.
   d. aspiration.

133. Amino acid–based solution for peritoneal dialysis is indicated for
   a. all patients.
   b. nutritionally compromised patients.
   c. diabetic patients.
   d. pregnant patients.

134. An upper chest presternal exit site for peritoneal dialysis may be indicated for
   a. patients wearing belt line above umbilicus.
   b. younger patients.
   c. patients who are morbidly obese.
   d. wheelchair-bound patients.

135. Mixing which of the following antibiotics with penicillin in the same dialysis solution bag is contraindicated?
   a. Vancomycin.
   b. Cefazolin.
   c. Ceftazidime.
   d. Gentamicin.

136. For what duration is vancomycin stable in dialysate stored at room temperature?
   a. 4 days.
   b. 7 days.
   c. 14 days.
   d. 28 days.

137. A patient on peritoneal dialysis tells the nurse that one of the employees at the patient's company has offered to give the patient a kidney in exchange for $100,000. The nurse should advise the patient that
   a. the employee may not be a match.
   b. it is illegal to buy or sell an organ.
   c. the employee should come for compatibility testing.
   d. the patient should keep the financial arrangement secret.

138. An 18-year-old female patient with CAPD has become increasingly withdrawn and is reluctant to be seen in public unless wearing a large coat. The patient is most likely experiencing
    a. body image disturbance.
    b. activity intolerance.
    c. ineffective thermoregulation.
    d. ineffective coping.

139. Considering the peritoneal equilibrium test (PET), patients in which of the following transporter categories would be expected to have the highest 4-hour dialysate to plasma creatinine, urea, and sodium (D/PCr, PUr, and PNa) values?
    a. Low transporters.
    b. Low-average transporters.
    c. High-average transporters.
    d. High transporters.

140. Which of the following diffuses from peritoneal capillary blood into peritoneal fluid during peritoneal dialysis?
    a. Glucose.
    b. Calcium.
    c. Bicarbonate.
    d. Potassium.

141. A patient with CAPD has decreased effluent volumes of dialysate and increased weight gain without peripheral edema. Physical examination shows an asymmetric protuberant abdomen. The most likely cause is
    a. abdominal wall leak.
    b. peri-catheter leak.
    c. hydrothorax.
    d. peritonitis.

142. If an infection occurs in an arteriovenous graft, the patient is at increased risk of
    a. hemorrhage.
    b. dialysis dementia.
    c. fluoride intoxication.
    d. hyperglycemia.

143. If a patient has active infectious tuberculosis and has been receiving hemodialysis, the treatments should be
    a. changed to peritoneal dialysis until the patient is not infectious.
    b. continued in an isolation room with negative air flow.
    c. continued in a standard isolation room.
    d. withheld until antitubercular medications started.

144. If a hemodialysis patient presents with shaking chills, high fever, myalgia, hypotension, nausea, and vomiting, the most likely causative agent is
    a. gram-negative bacteria.
    b. gram-positive bacteria.
    c. endotoxin.
    d. nontubercular Mycobacterium.

Section Description: Lee Case Questions

Darlene Lee, a 38-year-old woman with ESKD, is scheduled to begin hemodialysis and is scheduled to have an AV fistula created.

145. The physician carries out vessel mapping on Ms. Lee. The purpose of "vessel mapping" is to ensure
   a. the surgeon has completed the AV fistula properly.
   b. the blood flow distal to the AV fistula is adequate.
   c. the blood flow proximal to the AV fistula is adequate.
   d. the surgeon will find adequate vessels for the AV fistula.

146. During the first week of treatment with a new AV fistula, the initial blood flow rate is usually
   a. 400 to 450 mL/min.
   b. 250 to 300 mL/min
   c. 200 to 250 mL/min.
   d. 300 to 350 mL/min.

147. When determining if a new AV fistula is maturing, the 3 factors to assess by palpation are the
   a. thrill, vessel growth, and vessel firmness.
   b. pulse, sensitivity, and vessel growth.
   c. incision, pulse, and vessel growth.
   d. incision, vessel growth and pulse.

148. A week after Ms. Lee has an AV fistula created in the lower arm, she is referred to physical therapy for exercises to help mature the fistula. Exercises that she is advised to do likely include
   a. swinging the arm in circles.
   b. bicep curls.
   c. hammer curls.
   d. ball squeeze.

149. During the first week of treatment with a new AV fistula, the initial needle size is usually
   a. #14 gauge.
   b. #15 gauge.
   c. #17 gauge.
   d. #18 gauge.

150. With an AV fistula, cannulation should be done at an angle of
   a. 15° to 25°.
   b. 25° to 35°.
   c. 45°.
   d. 45° to 60°.

151. According to one element of the "Rule of 6s," an AV fistula is considered successful if it
   a. is 6 inches long.
   b. is 0.06 cm below the skin surface.
   c. has a 60 mL/min blood flow rate.
   d. is 0.6 cm wide.

152. Ms. Lee has little residual urine volume. According to the KDOQI, the minimum hemodialysis session length for a patient with little residual urine volume is
   a. 3 hours, 3 times a week.
   b. 4 hours, 3 times a week.
   c. 2 hours, 4 times a week.
   d. 4 hours, 2 times a week.

153. Ms. Lee's PTH level has increased. After initiation of calcitriol treatment for elevated PTH level, the patient's calcium level is 10.5 mg/dL. The appropriate response is to
   a. increase calcitriol dose by 25%.
   b. decrease calcitriol dose by 25%.
   c. decrease calcitriol dose by 50%.
   d. hold the calcitriol.

Section Description: Yager Case Questions

Samantha Yager, a 28-year-old woman on hemodialysis, has had a prosthetic arteriovenous graft implanted.

154. Maturation of a prosthetic arteriovenous graft usually takes
   a. 1 to 2 weeks.
   b. 3 to 6 weeks.
   c. 1 to 2 months.
   d. 2 to 4 month.

155. If routine heparin is administered with an initial bolus and subsequent infusion for anticoagulation while Ms. Yager is undergoing hemodialysis, the correct administration is
   a. inject bolus into arterial line, flush with saline, and then infuse heparin into venous line.
   b. inject bolus into venous line, flush with saline, and then infuse heparin into arterial line.
   c. inject bolus into venous line, flush with saline, and then infuse heparin into venous line
   d. inject bolus into arterial line, flush with saline, and then infuse heparin into arterial line.

156. After Ms. Yager receives the initial heparin bolus for hemodialysis, when should dialysis be initiated?
   a. Immediately.
   b. 1 to 2 minutes.
   c. 3 to 5 minutes.
   d. 5 to 8 minutes.

157. Routine heparin should generally be administered during hemodialysis to maintain an ACT level of baseline plus
   a. 20%.
   b. 40%.
   c. 60%.
   d. 80%.

158. The nurse is teaching Ms. Yager, who still urinates, to manage fluid intake with a base of 1000 mL intake per day. If the patient urinates 500 mL in a 24-hour period, how much fluid is the patient allowed the following day?
   a. 1500 mL.
   b. 1400 mL.
   c. 1250 mL.
   d. 1000 mL.

159. Five minutes after initiation of a hemodialysis treatment, Ms. Yager complains of dyspnea, generalized itching, tingling about the mouth, and feeling faint. The patient has periorbital edema, and hives are evident. The nurse should immediately call for help and
   a. decrease the blood flow rate.
   b. increase the ultrafiltration rate.
   c. provide oxygen.
   d. clamp all lines and stop dialysis.

Section Description: Mayer Case Questions

Sarah Mayer, a 26-year-old woman, develops hematuria, peripheral and pulmonary edema, hypertension, azotemia, and proteinuria, and is diagnosed with acute glomerulonephritis. The patient's BUN and serum creatinine levels are increased. The patient complains of headache, flank pain, and general malaise.

160. Ms. Mayer also presents with a malar rash, arthralgias, and oral lesions. Which disorder should be suspected as the precipitating factor for the acute glomerulonephritis?
   a. Rheumatoid arthritis.
   b. Systemic lupus erythematosus (SLE).
   c. Wegener granulomatosis.
   d. Renal cancer.

161. Based on these findings (including the malar rash, arthralgias, and oral lesions), in addition to a nephrologist, the patient may require consultation with a(n)
   a. oncologist.
   b. hematologist.
   c. immunologist.
   d. rheumatologist.

Section Description: Infection Case Questions

Two patients treated at a dialysis center have recently developed bloodstream infections. As a result, the staff members are reviewing infection control procedures and trying to identify and eliminate the underlying cause.

162. The greatest risk of bacteremia is associated with which type of vascular access?
   a. Primary arteriovenous fistula.
   b. Arteriovenous graft (biologic).
   c. Dialysis catheter.
   d. Arteriovenous graft (prosthetic).

163. The 3 bloodborne pathogens that pose the most risk for hemodialysis patients are
    a. hepatitis A, hepatitis B, and hepatitis C.
    b. hepatitis B, hepatitis C, and HIV.
    c. hepatitis B, Ebola, and HIV.
    d. hepatitis B, hepatitis D, and HIV.

164. According to the NQF criteria, when calculating the Standardized Infection Ratio (SIR) of bloodstream infections (BSIs) for patients treated in an ambulatory hemodialysis center, which data would be used for the numerator?
    a. The number of positive blood cultures drawn from outpatients of an ambulatory hemodialysis center or within 1 day of their hospitalization.
    b. The number of patients treated in the ambulatory hemodialysis center on the first 2 working days of the month.
    c. The number of both the patients treated in the ambulatory hemodialysis center and the patients treated with home dialysis.
    d. The number of patients with positive blood cultures drawn as outpatients only.

165. The staff reviews skin prep procedures. Which of the following antiseptics used for skin prep for a fistula site has the broadest spectrum antibacterial activity?
    a. Povidone iodine.
    b. Isopropyl alcohol 70%.
    c. Chlorhexidine gluconate 2%.
    d. Hydrogen peroxide.

166. The entire water system is examined to determine if it could be a factor in the infections. The purpose of a break tank or reduced pressure zone valve in the water system is to
    a. ensure adequate water supply.
    b. sterilize the water supply.
    c. decrease water pressure.
    d. prevent backflow.

167. While a patient is undergoing hemodialysis, chloramine testing should be conducted every
    a. hour.
    b. 2 hours.
    c. 4 hours.
    d. 5 hours.

168. The last component of the water processing system before the distribution loop should be a(n)
    a. ultrafilter.
    b. ultraviolet light.
    c. reverse osmosis device.
    d. deionizer.

169. Fluoride contamination of water used for hemodialysis may result in
    a. hemolysis.
    b. ventricular fibrillation.
    c. anemia.
    d. encephalopathy.

170. Which of the following contaminants of water used for dialysis may result in dialysis dementia?

   a. Zinc.
   b. Chloramine.
   c. Copper.
   d. Aluminum.

171. The external surface of the hemodialysis machine should be cleaned and disinfected at least

   a. every 8 hours.
   b. every 24 hours.
   c. after every patient.
   d. after every 2 patients.

172. When checking the water temperature in the water system, the temperature is recorded at 78 °F (25.5 °C). In order for the reverse osmosis (RO) equipment that is part of the water treatment system to work properly, the water temperature must be maintained at

   a. 74 °F to 76 °F (23.3 °C to 24.4 °C).
   b. 77 °F to 82 °F (25 °C to 28 °C).
   c. 83 °F to 86 °F (28.3 °C to 30 °C).
   d. 87 °F to 90 °F (30.5 °C to 32.2 °C).

Section Description: Walker Case Questions

Stephanie Walker is a 20-year-old college student with chronic kidney disease.

173. Ms. Walker has required frequent hospitalizations because of nonadherence to her treatment plan. The best approach to take with the patient is to

   a. point out how the patient has caused the hospitalizations.
   b. ask the patient how the nurse can help her better manage her condition.
   c. suggest that the patient needs to act in a more mature manner.
   d. advise the patient that she may benefit from psychological counseling.

174. Ms. Walker questions whether she will be able to have children. A patient of childbearing age with which of the following kidney diseases may be referred to a genetics counselor when considering pregnancy?

   a. Chronic pyelonephritis.
   b. Polycystic kidney disease (PKD).
   c. Glomerulonephritis.
   d. Nephrotic syndrome.

175. The nurse feels a special friendship toward Ms. Walker, who reminds the nurse of a close family member. The nurse should deal with this by

   a. acknowledging the feeling.
   b. asking for reassignment.
   c. avoiding the patient when possible.
   d. spending extra time with the patient.

Answer Key and Explanations

Section Description: Parker Case Questions

1. A: If a hemodialysis patient routinely experiences hypotensive episodes near the end of a session with malaise, muscle cramps, and dizziness after dialysis, the most likely cause is that the dry weight is set too low. If these symptoms occur, then the patient's dry weight may need to be adjusted. If the dry weight (the optimal post-dialysis weight) is set too high, the patient may experience fluid overload after dialysis, resulting in peripheral edema and/or pulmonary edema with subsequent ingestion of fluids.

2. B: Generally, the optimal dialysate flow rate should be 1.5 to 2 times the blood flow rate. The standard dialysate flow rate is 500 mL/min, but this may be increased to 800 mL/min for select patients; studies indicate little benefit above 600 mL/min. Increasing the time of dialysis rather than the dialysate flow rate may confer more benefit. The dialysis dose is affected by numerous other factors, such as the dialyzer's mass transfer area coefficient.

3. D: According to the National Kidney Foundation Kidney Disease Outcomes Quality Initiative (NKF KDOQI) guidelines, the minimum target spKt/V (single pool Kt/V) dose for patients receiving hemodialysis is 1.4 because the minimum dose for the patient is 1.2, but because there is a coefficient of variation among patients of 0.1 Kt/V units, the target dose is slightly higher to ensure the dose does not fall below 1.2. K refers to the dialyzer clearance of urea, t refers to the time/duration of dialysis, and V refers to the volume of body fluid (urea clearance area); the spKt/V is used to determine the adequacy of dialysis.

4. C: According to KDOQI guidelines, the dialysis dose for patients on hemodialysis should be monitored at least once monthly, sampling both pre-dialysis and post-dialysis BUNs. The blood samples for the BUNs should be collected at the same session. These values are then used to calculate the urea reduction ratio (URR) and spKt/V. To ensure accuracy, the proper sampling techniques must be followed carefully. Some variation in results is common, so averaging 3 monthly spKt/V values is often done before adjusting the dialysis prescription.

5. C: If the patient is receiving hemodialysis with a dialyzer with an ultrafiltration coefficient (K_{UF}) of 10 and a transmembrane pressure (TMP) of 100 mm Hg, the patient should lose 1000 mL of fluid per hour of treatment. Transmembrane pressure refers to the average difference in pressure from the blood side of the membrane to the dialysate side (blood side minus dialysate side pressure). The ultrafiltration coefficient (K_{UF}) (mL/h/mm Hg) is multiplied by the TMP:

- 10 (mL/h/mm Hg) × 100 (mm Hg) = 1000 mL/h

6. B: If a hemodialysis patient has a dialyzer clearance rate of 250 mL/min with a 4-hour (240-minute) treatment, the total volume of blood cleared is 60 L:

- 250 mL × 240 min = 60,000 mL or 60 L.

This clearance rate is used to calculate the Kt/V dose. The V refers to the total volume of fluid in the body, usually about 60% by weight; if a patient weighs 70 kg, the volume of water in the body is 70 × 0.6 = 42 L.

- Kt = 250 × 240 = 60 L
- V = 70 × 0.6 = 42.
- Kt/V = 60/42 = 1.4

7. B: When drawing a post-dialysis blood sample for BUN, one method is to slow the blood flow rate to 100 mL/min for 15 seconds before sampling because this duration of time is sufficient for unrecirculated blood to reach below the sampling port. As an alternative, the dialysate flow can be stopped for 3 minutes (or decreased to the minimum level if the equipment does not allow stopping the flow). This period of time is generally sufficient to stabilize the dialysate outlet BUN level with the blood inlet BUN level.

8. C: The target for serum ferritin for patients on hemodialysis is ≥200 ng/mL. Adults with normal kidney function usually are not diagnosed with iron deficiency anemia if their serum ferritin level is >15 ng/mL. However, the targets are higher with patients with chronic kidney disease because the inflammation associated with kidney disease increases the level of serum ferritin, so ≥100 ng/mL is recommended as the target for patients with chronic kidney disease and ≥200 ng/mL for patients on hemodialysis.

9. C: Albumin is a protein that is critically important for fluid balance in the body and is a measure of nutritional status in patients with grade 5 kidney failure (ESKD). Low serum albumin levels increase the risk of mortality, especially if the level falls below 3.5 g/dL. While albumin levels may vary (the value is generally between 3.6 and 5 g/dL), patients on hemodialysis should maintain serum albumin levels >4 g/dL to ensure levels do not fall below the safety margin.

Section Description: Bell Case Questions

10. D: If the partner of a patient with ESKD has volunteered as a living donor, the first concern when evaluating the donor is the person's psychological status. If the patient does not pass this assessment, further assessment is unnecessary. When a family member or partner is involved, it is very important to ascertain if there is a history of domestic abuse or circumstances that suggest coercion. The potential donor should be assessed for a history of psychiatric or psychological disorders as well as a history of substance abuse.

11. B: The information gleaned during a psychiatric consultation that is most likely to be a contraindication for kidney transplant is a history of nonadherence to treatment regimen. If the patient was unable to adhere to treatment during kidney failure, the patient is likely to encounter problems after transplantation, when following the treatment regimen is critical. Many patients have a history of psychiatric disorders, but this alone is not a contraindication, nor is a history of substance abuse. Many patients have a history of unemployment because of having to cope with a chronic illness.

12. B: Following kidney transplantation, fluids must be administered for both maintenance and replacement. Insensible loss is approximately 30 mL/h and is usually replaced with dextrose 5% in water, while other fluid losses, such as from urinary output and NG drainage, are commonly replaced with one-half normal saline. IV fluids are used to help control urinary output; if urinary output is low, the patient may be administered a bolus of 0.5 to 1 L of normal saline. Electrolytes are generally provided, if needed, in a separate infusion.

13. D: In the immediate postoperative period after kidney transplantation, the physician should be notified if urinary output is less than 60 mL/h for 2 consecutive hours, more than 300 mL/h for 4 hours, or more than 500 mL/h for 2 consecutive hours. Urinary output must be carefully monitored to assess kidney function and to determine the amount of replacement IV fluids required.

14. B: Kidney rejection within hours of transplantation is classified as hyperacute. Types of rejection include:

- Hyperacute: This can occur within a few minutes or hours of transplantation and results from anti-donor antibodies and complement system activation.
- Accelerated: This may occur within days of transplantation and involves reactivation of sensitized T cells.
- Acute: This may occur within days up to a number of weeks and involves primary activation of T cells.
- Chronic: This form develops over a period of months to years and involves multiple factors, both immunologic and nonimmunologic.

15. A: Cyclosporine, an immunosuppressive agent used to prevent kidney rejection after transplantation, can be especially nephrotoxic, so kidney function must be monitored carefully during administration. Nephrotoxicity increases with a number of drug-drug interactions (such as with NSAIDs, ranitidine, and many antibiotics), so patients should be advised to always consult with the physician before taking any medications, including OTC. Patients should also avoid St. John's wort, alfalfa sprouts, and grapefruit.

16. A: When a patient is discharged after kidney transplantation, the nurse should ensure the patient understands that the primary measures to determine the health of the kidney are serum creatinine and urinary output. Patients should keep a log of urinary output and should be aware of their serum creatinine levels, so that if patients see local physicians who are less familiar with kidney transplants, the patients can alert the physicians to levels of concern. Any increase of 25% or more in the serum creatinine requires immediate assessment of kidney function.

Section Description: Woods Case Questions

17. D: The most common cause of acute kidney injury (AKI) in critically ill patients, especially elderly patients, is sepsis because sepsis results in hemodynamic instability and hypoperfusion. Therefore, the first-line treatment is fluid resuscitation with intravenous fluids; however, because of increased vascular permeability resulting from inflammation, the fluid may move into the interstitial (third) space. Vasopressors are often used to combat hypotension, but they may also increase vascular resistance in the kidney microvasculature.

18. C: If a patient with acute renal failure has increasing peripheral edema and pulmonary congestion with decreased urinary output, the medication of choice is likely a loop diuretic, such as furosemide. Studies indicate that loop diuretics do not improve outcomes for patients who are severely ill with AKI; however, the diuretics increase urinary output and may relieve edema and pulmonary congestion in patients with heart failure, so they are frequently prescribed.

19. A: In a patient with AKI, if ECG telemetry shows peaked T waves and widening of the QRS interval, signs that may lead to ventricular tachycardia or fibrillation, these changes may be indicative of hyperkalemia. Other indications of hyperkalemia (>4.5 mEq/L) are irritability, anxiety, nausea and vomiting, weakness, abdominal cramping, and numbness and tingling of the fingertips and around the mouth. With AKI, levels may increase to ≥6 mEq/L in a short period of time.

20. B: If a patient with AKI and anuria has a potassium level that has increased from 4.5 to 6 mmol/L in a short time, the most likely temporary emergent treatment is insulin (10 units regular) and glucose (50 mL of dextrose 50% solution) per infusion as this causes the potassium to move from the serum and into the cells. Diuretics may be given to decrease potassium but only if the patient is producing adequate urine. Sodium polystyrene sulfonate (Kayexalate) or dialysis may be used as permanent methods to reduce potassium levels.

21. B: In a patient with acute kidney injury, if the serum creatinine (a byproduct of muscle metabolism) increases from 0.75 to 1.5 mg/dL, the nurse expects that the GFR will decrease by 50%. Normal creatinine ranges from 0.5 to 1.2 mg/dL (45 to 107 micromole/L). The potential critical value is greater than 7.4 mg/dL in nondialytic patients. Chronic renal insufficiency occurs with creatinine of 1.5 to 3 mg/dL with renal failure present at greater than 3 mg/dL.

Section Description: Rule Case Questions

22. B: Hemolytic uremic syndrome (HUS), a complication of *E. coli* (O157:H7) infection, is characterized by the triad of (1) acute renal failure, (2) microangiopathic hemolytic anemia, and (3) thrombocytopenia. HUS is most common in children younger than 5 years or older adults. Bacterial toxins from the *E. coli* enter the bloodstream from the intestines, causing damage to small vessels in the kidneys and sometimes other organs as well. Urinary output decreases as the diarrhea progresses.

23. D: Initial therapy for HUS usually includes intravenous fluids to maintain fluid and electrolyte balance. Antibiotics should generally be avoided because they may stimulate the release of extra toxin; however, antibiotics may be necessary if the patient develops sepsis. Antimotility agents increase the risk that the *E. coli* infection will progress to HUS and they should be avoided as well. Plasmapheresis may be used to remove antibodies from the blood. ACE inhibitors may help prevent permanent kidney damage.

24. A: With HUS, the part of the kidney that is damaged is the glomeruli. Toxins destroy platelets, and clotting time increases. Red blood cells fragment when they flow through areas of thrombi. The glomeruli are damaged when they become obstructed with damaged platelets and red blood cells, interfering with the kidneys' ability to filter waste products. About half of the patients with HUS progress to acute kidney failure and some may require ongoing dialysis or kidney transplant. About a third of those who develop kidney failure have delayed abnormalities of kidney function later in life.

Section Description: Kim Case Questions

25. A: If a 58-year old patient with type 2 diabetes and ESKD has been treated with CAPD for 2 years and develops numerous painful firm brown nodules on both lower legs with some nodules eroding and becoming necrotic, as well as mottled skin and decreased sensation, the most likely cause is calcific uremic arteriolopathy (CUA). CUA is a life-threatening disorder associated with kidney failure in which arterioles become calcified and result in necrosis of the tissue. It is more common in patients with diabetic comorbidity, and incidence is higher in females than males.

26. D: The treatment that is most commonly used to treat CUA is IV or intraperitoneal (IP) sodium thiosulfate. Biopsies carry a high risk of mortality but may help to guide treatment. Surgical debridement is contraindicated. Corticosteroids and immunosuppressive agents may worsen the condition. Some studies have indicated that patients on PD seem to be at higher risk of CUA than those on HD, perhaps because phosphate levels tend to be higher with PD. Secondary hyperparathyroidism is also an increased risk factor because of resultant hyperphosphatemia.

Section Description: Anders Case Questions

27. C: A patient with diabetes mellitus (either type 1 or type 2) and chronic kidney disease should generally have a target HbA_{1c} of less than 7%, but the A_{1c} may be individualized for the patient with type 2 diabetes. Additionally, KDOQI guidelines suggest that the target may need to be adjusted upward for patients who tend to be hypoglycemic or have multiple comorbidities. Good glycemic control can slow progression of kidney disease.

28. B: In a diabetic patient with chronic kidney failure, glycosuria is unreliable as an estimation of hyperglycemia because the damaged nephrons may be inconsistent in excreting excess glucose. Normally, urine does not contain glucose; however, if there is an excess load of glucose, it may not all be reabsorbed. With normal kidney function, glycosuria usually occurs when serum glucose levels are greater than 180 mg/dL, but with kidney failure, this may vary widely.

29. A: As chronic kidney disease progresses, the endocrinologic change that can result in higher risk of fractures is hyperparathyroidism. As kidney function declines, less vitamin D is converted to its active form, so less calcium is absorbed, resulting in hypocalcemia. As a compensatory measure, the parathyroid gland secretes increased amounts of parathyroid hormone (PTH) to stimulate demineralization and release increased amounts of the calcium and phosphate from the bones, resulting in weakened bony matrix.

30. B: According to KDIGO guidelines, treatment with an erythropoiesis-stimulating agent (ESA) for anemia associated with chronic kidney disease should not be initiated until the hemoglobin level falls to less than 10 g/dL. Anemia tends to worsen as the kidneys fail, resulting in anemia because of deficiency of erythropoietin or iron; however, using an ESA to increase the hemoglobin level to 13 g/dL shows no benefit and may increase risk of complications. It also has no effect on the progression of kidney disease, so only partial correction is generally done.

31. D: A patient with chronic kidney disease must have dialysis or transplantation in order to survive when kidney function falls below 10% to 15%, the indication for ESKD (stage 5 kidney failure). Prior to this, CKD may be managed with some combination of fluid restriction, dietary sodium restriction, and medications (such as ARBs, phosphate binders, and diuretics), although the patient's quality of life may gradually deteriorate as the GFR falls because of increasing physical limitations and complications.

32. A: Dialysis is usually started when a patient with uremia has a GFR (MDRD equation) of <15 mL/min/1.73 m². Stages of chronic kidney disease are as follows:

18. GRF remains relatively normal (≥90 mL/min/1.73 m²)
19. GFR decreasing (60 to 89 mL/min/1.73 m²) with mild kidney damage and focus on assessing progression
20. GFR further decreases (30 to 59 mL/min/1.73 m²) with moderate kidney damage and focus on evaluating and treating complications
21. GFR decreases (15 to 29 mL/min/1.73 m²) with severe kidney damage and focus on preparing for dialysis
22. Kidney failure with GRF <15 mL/min/1.73 m² and a candidate for dialysis and/or kidney transplant

Section Description: Aiken Case Questions

33. D: When assisting a surgeon with stencil-based preoperative mapping for insertion of a peritoneal dialysis catheter, the patient should be initially positioned supine so that the abdomen can be easily visualized and the stencil placed in various positions that are appropriate for different catheters and the exit sites marked with a marking pen. Then, the patient is assisted to sitting and standing positions so that the surgeon can evaluate the exit sites in relation to skin folds, creases, and the belt line. When an exit site is selected, the mapping is completed.

34. A: Prior to surgical placement of a catheter for peritoneal dialysis, the recommended antibiotic prophylaxis is generally a first-generation cephalosporin. Vancomycin is also frequently used, but the issue of antibiotic resistance should be considered carefully and balanced against benefits of vancomycin. Usually 1 dose of antibiotic is given at the time of the catheter insertion. A double-cuff catheter is recommended because of lower rates of infection and other site complications.

35. C: If a culture of the catheter exit site is positive for *Staphylococcus aureus* but there is no erythema or purulent discharge, the most likely cause of the positive culture is colonization, which frequently occurs within a short time after insertion of the catheter. Colonization is a form of contamination that can lead to more serious infections because colonized bacteria are more resistant to antibiotics. Erythema, by itself, is not always indicative of an infection while purulent discharge is.

36. B: While not used in a hospital environment, a heating pad may be used to warm dialysate solution in the home environment. Maintaining a stable temperature can be difficult and warming may take a prolonged period of time. The heating pad should have an automatic shut-off time to prevent overheating (usually about 2 hours). With this method of heating, it is especially important to check the temperature of the solution prior to instillation. Other methods used include warming cabinets and microwave ovens (not recommended but frequently used).

37. B: Once a dialysate bag is heated, the temperature can be assessed by folding the bag over and enclosing an electronic thermometer. The temperature of the dialysate should be at body temperature (37 °C) because instilling room temperature dialysate may result in chills and lowering of the body temperature. The bag should be rotated to mix the solution thoroughly before measuring temperature in case hot spots are present, especially if the dialysate was heated in a microwave oven.

38. C: With CAPD, the number of exchanges in 24 hours is usually 4 to 5 with 3 to 4 done during the daytime hours (every 4 to 6 hours) and 1 longer exchange done during the night. During the daytime, drainage usually takes about 20 minutes. The dwell time during the night is extended to 8 to 10 hours to allow the patient to sleep. The dextrose concentration of the overnight dwell may be higher than that used during the day because of the longer duration.

39. C: With CAPD, the volume of dialysate retained in the peritoneal cavity (dwell) at all times in adults is usually approximately ≤2 L. Exchanges are usually carried out every 3 to 4 hours during the day. The dialysate is instilled in about 10 minutes, during which the patient may sit, stand, or lie down. After instillation, the catheter is clamped until the prescribed dwell time is completed and then drained.

Section Description: Maddox Case Questions

40. B: When teaching a patient with kidney failure and hemodialysis to manage fluid balance, the nurse advises the patient that a 1 kg (2.2 lb) increase in weight in 24 hours is approximately equivalent to fluid retention of 1 L. Patients should be advised to monitor intake and output and take daily weights. Patients' "dry" weight should be estimated every 3 to 6 weeks in order to help to estimate weight gain related to fluids. Weight gained between dialysis treatments should not exceed 5% of the dry weight estimate.

41. A: If a patient on hemodialysis has been advised to avoid foods high in phosphorus, foods that should be limited include dairy products. Other foods and beverages that are high in phosphorous include beer, ale, colas, chocolate, high-protein meats (liver, organ meats), oysters, sardines, dried beans and peas, nuts, seeds, whole grains, and wheat germ and bran. Normal phosphorous level is 2.5 to 4.5 mg/dL. Lowering phosphorous levels helps to increase absorption of calcium.

42. D: If a patient on hemodialysis has been prescribed sevelamer hydrochloride as a phosphate binder, the patient should be advised to take this medication with meals. Because sevelamer hydrochloride may bind to other medications and decrease their bioavailability, other drugs should be given an hour before sevelamer or 3 hours after. The dosage of sevelamer should be adjusted to maintain a phosphorous level of 3.5 to 5.5 mg/dL. Calcium, bicarbonate, and chloride levels should be monitored as well as phosphorous.

43. B: If a patient who usually drinks 2 cups of caffeinated coffee daily has headaches during hemodialysis, the patient should be advised to drink a cup of strong coffee with treatment to compensate for lack of caffeine loss during hemodialysis. The patient is likely experiencing caffeine withdrawal. As an alternative, the patient can transition to decaffeinated beverages. Taking acetaminophen at the beginning of treatment may help to prevent or control the headaches.

Section Description: Independent Questions, Group 1

44. C: If the patient cannot tolerate contrast for a CT and needs an MRI to evaluate a mass on his kidney, cancelling the MRI is not a viable solution. When patients are very claustrophobic, reassuring them or advising them to practice relaxation is not likely to be effective, so the best solution is likely to contact the physician and request an order for a sedative. Generally, when patients require sedation to relieve anxiety, alprazolam (Xanax) is the medication of choice and is usually administered immediately before the procedure.

45. B: The first indication of renal cancer is often painless hematuria, which may be intermittent or continuous. Hematuria may also present as frank bleeding or be evident microscopically. Renal cancer is often essentially asymptomatic until it has metastasized. Only about 10% of patients present with the classic signs of renal cancer: hematuria, flank pain, and palpable mass. Because of this, renal cancers are often found incidentally. Patients may develop flank pain as the tumor increases in size and presses against adjacent structures.

46. C: For a patient with ESKD diagnosed with tuberculosis, both isoniazid and rifampin can usually be given at 100% the normal dose. However, ethambutol, pyrazinamide, and rifabutin dosages should be reduced to 50% of the normal dose. Incidence of tuberculosis is higher in the patients with chronic kidney disease and patients on dialysis than in the general population because of reduced cellular immunity associated with kidney failure. While protocols vary, patients often receive isoniazid, rifampicin, and pyrazinamide (or ethambutol) for 2 months and then isoniazid and rifampicin for 10 to 18 months.

47. C: According to the RIFLE (Risk, Injury, Failure, Loss of kidney function, ESKD) criteria for acute kidney dysfunction, urinary output indicative of kidney failure is <0.3 mL/kg/h for 24 hours. Other indications include serum creatinine 3 times normal or serum creatinine of ≥4 mg/dL with an acute rise in serum creatinine of ≥0.5 mg/dL. The RIFLE criteria are used to determine the risk of critically ill patients developing acute kidney injury (AKI). The first 3 categories (RIF) indicate increasing severity of disease and the last 2 (LE) indicate outcome criteria.

48. A: If a patient's cardiac output decreases, resulting in arterial hypoperfusion with reduced blood flow to the kidneys, the nurse expects lab results to show increased BUN because the reduced blood flow reduces glomerular filtration and urinary output, allowing the BUN to increase. If perfusion is restored quickly, then the kidneys may not have permanent damage; but, if perfusion is not restored quickly, significant irreversible renal damage may occur. This type of prerenal AKI is common in patients with critical illness.

49. D: Tumor lysis syndrome is an example of an intrarenal cause of AKI. AKI may be prerenal, intrarenal, or postrenal, depending on the cause:

- Prerenal: extended hypotension (sepsis, vasodilation), low cardiac output (heart failure, cardiogenic shock), volume depletion (hemorrhage, dehydration), and renovascular thrombosis.
- Intrarenal: kidney ischemia, endogenous toxins (rhabdomyolysis, tumor lysis syndrome), exogenous toxins (contrast dyes, nephrotoxic drugs).
- Postrenal: obstruction (ureters, bladder, urethra).

50. B: Many commonly used medications are nephrotoxic, especially if taken in large amounts. Drugs that may cause tubular cell toxicity include aminoglycosides, antiretrovirals, contrast dye, zoledronate, and amphotericin B. Because the proximal tubular cells actively concentrate and reabsorb glomerular filtrate, the cells are exposed to toxic elements. Other pathogenic mechanisms include alterations in intraglomerular hemodynamics, inflammation, crystal nephropathy, rhabdomyolysis, and thrombotic microangiopathy.

51. A: Prior to a serum creatinine test, the patient should be advised to avoid excessive exercise because creatinine is a product of muscle metabolism, and excessive exercise may cause a sudden increase. About 98% of creatinine is in the muscles, and virtually all of it is excreted through the kidneys. Thus, if the kidney tubules are impaired, the serum creatinine level rises. Creatinine is monitored to determine if kidney function is stable, decreasing, or increasing.

52. C: The primary preventive measure to avoid contrast-induced nephrotoxic injury for a patient who must receive IV radiopaque contrast material despite chronic kidney dysfunction is IV normal saline. Hydration should be carried out aggressively both during the procedure and after. In some cases, patients may be able to hydrate orally by drinking several liters of water over 12 hours. Avoiding dehydration is critical. N-acetylcysteine and fenoldopam have not been shown to provide additional benefit, and studies on the benefit of adding sodium bicarbonate have been inconclusive.

53. D: African Americans are the ethnic group that is most at risk for development of kidney failure, accounting for about a third of the cases in the United States. African Americans have high rates of both hypertension and diabetes mellitus, both of which increase the risk of kidney damage. Other groups that have increased risk of kidney failure are Hispanic Americans (twice the risk of Caucasians), Asian Americans, Pacific Islanders, and Native Americans. These ethnic groups also have high rates of diabetes and hypertension.

54. C: Patients may be advised to fast for at least 4 hours prior to a CT of the kidney with IV iodinated contrast because patients may experience nausea and vomiting. These adverse effects usually last only for a few moments, but patients who have recently eaten food are more likely to vomit. Patients with chronic kidney disease are especially at risk for contrast-induced nephropathy and should have volume expansion before and after the CT either through oral or IV fluids.

55. B: The primary cause of nephrosclerosis is hypertension and diabetes. Nephrosclerosis results in hardening of the renal arteries and is a main cause of chronic kidney disease and ESKD. In younger adults, malignant nephrosclerosis occurs with significant hypertension and is more common in males than females. The impaired perfusion of the kidneys results in necrotic areas and fibrosis, leading to uremia. Benign nephrosclerosis may occur in older adults who have hypertension and atherosclerosis.

56. C: If shortly after admission for postinfectious acute glomerulonephritis the patient develops altered mental status, the most likely cause of this complication is hypertensive encephalopathy, which may occur with acute glomerulonephritis and is an emergent condition that requires immediate treatment with vasodilators/antihypertensives. Infections that may precipitate acute glomerulonephritis include group A beta-hemolytic streptococcal infection (usually pharyngitis) and numerous viral infections, including Epstein-Barr, hepatitis B, and HIV.

57. D: Prerenal kidney failure, associated with renal hypoperfusion, may result from volume depletion, which may be caused by severe dehydration, hemorrhage, diuresis (sometimes related to diuretics), vomiting, diarrhea, and NG suctioning. Other causes of prerenal failure include impaired cardiovascular functioning, such as may occur with MI, heart failure, cardiac dysrhythmias, and cardiogenic shock. Prerenal kidney failure may also result from marked vasodilation that occurs with sepsis, anaphylaxis, and antihypertensive medications.

58. A: Characteristic of acute prerenal kidney failure is sodium level of less than 20 mEq/L compared with greater than 40 mEq/L for intrarenal renal failure. BUN and serum creatinine are increased, similar to intrarenal kidney failure, while urinary output is decreased with prerenal and increased with intrarenal. Urine sediment is usually within normal parameters with a few hyaline casts with prerenal failure while abnormal casts and debris are common with intrarenal. Urine osmolality is more than 500 mOsm/L with prerenal failure and less than 350 mOsm/L with intrarenal. Specific gravity is increased with prerenal and low normal with intrarenal failure.

59. B: The obligatory urine output (minimal amount of urinary output) that is needed to filter normal metabolic waste products and remove them from the body is about 500 mL. Normal kidneys must be able to excrete urine ranging from very dilute to very concentrated, as this is necessary to regulate serum sodium and fluid balance. Kidneys normally excrete a solute load of 600 to 800 mOsm per day. The maximum capacity of the kidneys to concentrate urine is 1200 mOsm per liter, so if a patient has solute excretion of 600 mOsm (half his maximum capacity), the minimal urine output is 0.5 L (500 mL).

60. D: The medication that is nephrotoxic and should have baseline and follow-up BUN and serum creatinine monitored during administration is vancomycin. Numerous medications may be nephrotoxic, but medications with increased risk that require monitoring include aminoglycosides, gentamicin, tobramycin, cyclosporine, amphotericin B, and polymyxin B. ACE inhibitors should be discontinued or carefully monitored if serum creatinine levels are significantly elevated. Some diuretics commonly used in treatment of kidney failure, such as furosemide, may also have nephrotoxic properties.

61. A: With kidney disease, decreased specific gravity may result from volume excess and intrarenal acute kidney injury. Decreased specific gravity occurs when the kidneys are not able to adequately excrete solutes. Increased specific gravity, on the other hand, results from volume deficit, glycosuria, and proteinuria as well as prerenal acute kidney injury. Specific gravity is the measure of the water by weight in comparison to distilled water (which has a specific gravity of 1.000), so the more solutes in the urine, the greater the specific gravity. Normal values range from 1.005 to 1.03.

62. B: If a patient with kidney failure has an order for a sodium polystyrene sulfonate (Kayexalate) retention enema, the nurse expects that the patient is being treated for hyperkalemia (value greater than 5.5 mEq/L). Hyperkalemia is characterized by diarrhea, generalized muscle weakness, abdominal cramping, slurred speech, dyspnea, and paresthesia. ECG abnormalities, such as peaked T waves, may occur, increasing the risk of cardiac arrest if hyperkalemia is not promptly treated and reversed.

63. D: If a patient with acute renal failure is stabilizing and seems alert and responsive, but the nurse notes that the patient needs to have explanations for treatment and procedures repeated many times, the most likely reason is anxiety. Acute renal failure may cause severe anxiety because of the intensive treatment, including dialysis, that may be needed to stabilize the patient, and the patient may be inundated with information and decisions. Patients may have difficulty concentrating and remembering details.

Section Description: Evans Case Questions

64. B: For a patient undergoing peritoneal dialysis, when sending a sample of cloudy dialysate for culture and sensitivities, the minimal sample size is 10 mL. Ideally, the sample should be processed immediately, but if processing must be delayed, the sample can be stored at 4 °C for up to 6 hours. Only cloudy dialysate should be cultured, and incubation may require up to a week. Dialysate cultures are frequently negative in the presence of peritonitis, likely because of inadequate culture techniques.

65. D: Minimal diagnostic criteria for peritonitis in a patient undergoing peritoneal dialysis usually includes tenderness around the catheter site and purulent discharge as well as at least 2 of the following: abdominal pain, dialysate WBC greater than 100 cells/mm³ and 50 PMN leukocytes, cloudy dialysate, and positive culture or gram stain of the dialysate. Infections associated with peritoneal dialysis include exit-site infection (erythema, purulent and/or sanguinous drainage, tenderness, edema around exit site), subcutaneous tunnel infections (erythema, edema, purulent discharge, or cellulitis), and peritonitis.

66. A: If a patient is being treated for peritonitis and fibrinous clots are visible in the dialysis effluent, the treatment of choice is heparin, administered intraperitoneally. Fibrin formation is often associated with the onset of peritonitis but it may also occur occasionally as part of routine peritoneal dialysis. Small amounts of the heparin may be absorbed systemically but most is not. However, the heparin may cause a local reaction in which damage may occur to mesothelial cells. Heparin may interfere with the action of rifampin but is compatible with most antibiotics.

Section Description: Elmers Case Questions

67. D: Patients receiving hemodialysis should be advised to wash the access site with soap and water before coming for treatment. Because *Staphylococcus aureus* may colonize at the access site, poor hygiene increases the risk of infection, so patients should be advised of the importance of good hygiene and should be trained to bathe regularly and wash the access site daily and before hemodialysis treatments. Patients should also be advised to monitor healthcare personnel to ensure they are using proper aseptic techniques and proper handwashing.

68. A: If a patient on hemodialysis is pregnant and her blood pressure is 160/100 mm Hg when euvolemic, an acceptable medication to treat hypertension is labetalol. Atenolol is contraindicated because it is classified as pregnancy risk category D. Both ACE inhibitors and ARBs are associated with congenital abnormalities, including dysplastic kidneys, neonatal anuria, pulmonary hypoplasia, and skull ossification defects. Hydralazine can be given in addition to other medications but should not be used as a single agent.

69. D: In order to increase the chance that the patient on hemodialysis will deliver a viable infant, ideally the pregnant patient should be dialyzed more than 20 hours per week. Intensive dialysis has been shown to decrease premature delivery and increase live births; however, the optimal number of hours per week has not been established. One study showed that most infants survived when the mother had 48 hours of dialysis per week. Both increased PD and hemodialysis increase survival rates, but it is more difficult to increase the hours of PD.

70. B: When calculating the amount of that must be removed during dialysis, fluid to offset the patient's weight gain must be included (1 kg = 1000 mL). Added to this is the volume of saline used to prime the system, any medications added in liquid form, the saline used to clear the system at the completion of the treatment, and any fluids ingested during treatment. This would include fluids, such as coffee, water, ginger ale, or ice chips.

71. D: Patients undergoing hemodialysis should avoid vitamin A supplements because nonuremic patients with high levels of vitamin A may develop severe adverse effects, and vitamin A may cause anemia as well as abnormalities of calcium metabolism and lipids. Other supplements that should generally be avoided include vitamin E, beta-carotene, and retinol. Fat-soluble vitamins are not removed by dialysis and therefore should not be supplemented. Patients should receive supplements of folic acid and B vitamins because water-soluble vitamins are lost through dialysis.

Case Description: Shaw Case Questions

72. D: For a patient receiving APD with most dialysis occurring during the night, the best time to take a plasma sample to determine the urea level is mid-afternoon because this is usually in the middle of the non-cycling period. For patients receiving APD, the urea level is usually lowest in the early AM at the end of cycling and highest in the evening before cycling. For patients receiving CAPD, the urea levels stay fairly stable because dialysis is continuous, so serum can be obtained at any time during the day.

73. B: With APD, may be used rather than glucose solution for the long day dwell. Icodextrin is a polyglucose solution that induces ultrafiltration and is absorbed by the lymphatics at a slower rate than glucose, making it best suited for long dwells, such as the long nocturnal dwell with CAPD and the long daytime dwell with APD. It is not used for short dwells, as it is not more effective than glucose and is more costly. Icodextrin is generally restricted to only 1 long dwell daily.

74. C: With APD, the patient should expect to spend 8 to 10 nighttime hours cycling. The number of cycles per night may vary from 3 to 10 with various dwell times, usually beginning at about 10 PM and continuing until about 7 AM. A variety of different patterns may be used with APD:

- Day dry: night cycles with no daytime dwell.
- Long day dwell: night cycles with long daytime dwell.
- Morning dwell: night cycles with morning dwell until noon.
- Evening dwell: night cycles with evening dwell from 5 to 10 PM.

Section Description: Mayweather Case Questions

75. C: If a patient who has been treated for kidney failure with hemodialysis for 5 years has developed pain and stiffness in the joints, the most likely cause is amyloidosis. This typically occurs after about 5 years of treatments because hemodialysis is not able to adequately filter amyloid proteins out of the blood as effectively as healthy kidneys. Amyloid proteins build up in organs and in joints and tendons, and the deposits damage the joints. Treatment is palliative only; there is no effective treatment or cure.

76. D: If a patient with kidney failure complains of severe itching during and after hemodialysis despite taking a phosphate binder, diphenhydramine (Benadryl) is commonly prescribed and may relieve itching for some patients. Some patients also find relief from hydroxyzine (Atarax). Ultraviolet light exposure through direct sunlight or light box may also reduce itching. If itching is unremitting, some patients have part of their parathyroid glands removed to reduce the increased levels of parathyroid hormone, which may cause itching.

77. A: A primary advantage of home hemodialysis is the ability to do more frequent treatments. At hemodialysis centers, treatments are usually done for 3 to 4 hours three times a week; with home hemodialysis, the patient can take shorter daily treatments so there is less fluid and waste buildup in the body, lowering the risk of complications. Patients are able to schedule treatments at their own convenience, giving them more freedom to live their lives. While costs remain high, patients may save expenses related to travel, especially if the center is far away.

78. B: If using a combination chlorhexidine gluconate and alcohol skin prep (such as ChloraPrep) before cannulation, the skin contact time required is 30 seconds. Then, the prep should be allowed to dry thoroughly (up to 3 minutes on hairless skin) before cannulation. Alcohol prep used alone also should have skin contact of 30 seconds. Povidone iodine prep (such as Betadine), however, requires a longer contact time of at least 3 minutes.

79. D: The most important factor for creation of a buttonhole technique for hemodialysis is that the same cannulator does all treatments until the tunnel is established, and this can take up to 10 cannulations in patients who are good healers or 14 for patients who are slow healers, such as diabetic patients. Different cannulators may cause a cone-shaped tunnel. The original cannulator should carefully document the insertion site and the angle of insertion and should ideally supervise subsequent cannulators. When possible, patients should be taught to self-cannulate once the tunnel is well established.

80. C: If a patient on home hemodialysis has buttonhole tracks, after the area is cleansed and prepped for treatment, the next step is to use a scab picker/aseptic tweezers to remove the scabs that form over the opening of the tracts. Once these are removed, blunt needles are inserted into the tracks for the treatment. Using the treatment needle to remove scabs increases risk of infection. Buttonhole tracks form literal tunnels to the vein. The tunnels stay open, much like a pierced ear.

81. B: Following home dialysis for a patient with buttonhole tracks, the patient should be taught to apply firm pressure as the needles are removed and then to maintain the pressure for 5 to 10 minutes after, depending on how long it takes for a clot to form. Because the buttonhole tract is open, if the patient removes the needle without applying pressure with a gauze pad, blood will spurt freely out of the tracks.

82. C: If a patient's buttonhole access for hemodialysis frequently has long clots that are very difficult to remove, the most likely reason is failure to use the 2-finger hold for needle removal. It is important when removing the needle to apply pressure to both the opening into the skin and the opening into the fistula using 2 fingers, which should easily span both openings. If the opening into the fistula is not compressed, blood will leak into the tunnel, forming a large clot.

83. A: With buttonhole access sites, the cannulator should leave 1/16th to 1/8th inch of the needle exposed to prevent "hubbing." Hubbing occurs when the hub of the needle presses against the buttonhole access site or imbeds into the site, causing the opening to dilate and form a bowl shape, increasing the risk of infection. Because a larger clot may form within the hubbed area, the clot may be difficult to completely remove and the site is more difficult to clean. Additionally, hubbing may result in damage to the epithelial lining of the tunnel.

84. D: The most common predisposing factor for muscle cramping during hemodialysis is hypotension. Other factors may include hypovolemia, high ultrafiltration rate because of excessive weight gain, and low sodium dialysate. All of these factors may result in vasoconstriction and decreased perfusion to the muscles and cramping. Cramping is more likely to occur in the first weeks of dialysis. In some cases, cramping may be related to hypocalcemia.

85. C: Indications of clotting in the extracorporeal circuit include blood foaming followed by clot formations in the drip chamber and the venous trap. Other indications include blood that is very dark in color; shadows or black streaks in the dialyzer; teetering in the venous line segment past the dialyzer, preventing the blood from entering the venous chamber and causing it to flow back into the line segment; and clots in the inflow dialyzer header. Analyzing pressure readings may help to locate clots that are occlusive.

86. D: Foam in the venous blood line of a dialyzer may indicate air embolism. While an air embolism may be venous or arterial, venous is more common and may result from system leaks, insertion of central venous catheter, or air in dialysate. If the patient is seated, the air embolism may enter the cerebral circulation, causing severe neurological impairment. If the patient is lying down, the air embolism may enter the heart and lungs, resulting in cardiac arrhythmias and respiratory distress.

87. A: When a patient is using home hemodialysis, the purpose of teaching the patient to "snap and tap" the tubing and filter is to remove air bubbles. Once the filter and tubing are attached to the equipment, it is primed with normal saline, and this clears out the air, but some bubbles may remain, and snapping and tapping helps to move the bubbles. Some microbubbles may persist, but large bubbles pose a risk and should be removed. The filter should be checked carefully for streaking, which can indicate an air pocket. The snap and tap procedure may take 5 to 15 minutes.

Section Description: Jones Case Questions

88. C: The psychiatric disorder that is most common in patients with ESKD is depression, which may occur in 10% to 50% of patients on dialysis. One of the primary problems associated with depression is nonadherence because patients who are depressed may feel that compliance with treatment is pointless, or they may be suicidal and feel that they want to die. In fact, suicide rates are higher for dialysis patients than for the general population. Psychiatric problems affect about 10% of hospitalized patients with ESKD.

89. C: If a patient with ESKD is screened with the Beck Depression Inventory (BDI) and has a score of 20, this suggests moderate depression. This tool has 21 items that are scored from 0 (no problem) to 3 (severe). The higher the score, the more severe the depression. BDI is normed for adults between the ages of 17 and 80 years and is often used to screen patients with kidney disease. Scores:

- 0 to 9 no signs of depression
- 10 to 18 mild depression
- 19 to 29 moderate depression
- 30 to 63 severe depression

90. A: For a patient with ESKD, the dosage of an SSRI should be reduced by two-thirds. SSRIs pose an increased risk of bleeding and nausea and vomiting, symptoms that may occur with ESKD, so the patient must be monitored carefully. However, the SSRI may provide some additional benefit by decreasing incidence of postural and intradialytic hypotension because of improved vascular tone. The most common drug prescribed for ESKD patients is fluoxetine (usually 20 mg daily).

91. C: The purpose of a high-carbohydrate diet for a patient with kidney failure is to spare protein for growth and healing. Protein intake must be individualized so that the body's requirements for protein are met while preventing symptoms related to uremia. With a high-carbohydrate diet, the carbohydrates are burned to provide energy for the body while the protein is "spared." Patients may need to limit some high carbohydrate foods that are also high in potassium, so consultation with a nutritionist is an important part of dietary education.

Section Description: Independent Questions, Group 2

92. B: Femoral catheters for vascular access for hemodialysis should be left in place for no longer than 5 days. Femoral catheters are generally contraindicated because of the increased potential for complications and infections and should only be used for short periods in patients who are bedbound. While puncture of the femoral artery usually only results in a hematoma, with femoral access, dialysis should be heparin-free for at least the first 24 hours. Femoral access increases risk of vein thrombosis.

93. A: If a patient develops an infection of a primary AV fistula and requires more than 6 weeks of antibiotic treatment, subacute endocarditis should be suspected. Risk increases with the presence of a calcified valve, a common finding after about 5 years of dialysis treatments. Some patients may be treated solely with antibiotics, but others may require valve replacement because the valve has become so damaged. Commonly found causative agents include *Staphylococcus aureus* and MRSA.

94. D: For short-term central venous catheters (CVCs) in adults, the CDC recommends that transparent dressings be changed every 7 days unless they become loosened and require more frequent changes. Gauze dressings should be changed every 2 days. Following the insertion of the CVC, the CDC recommends the initial dressing be changed only every 7 days until the exit site is well healed because more frequent dressing changes increase the risk of contamination of the exit site and infection.

95. B: If a patient with acute tubular necrosis is receiving hemodialysis, the phase of the disease that may be obscured is diuresis. Typically, output during this phase is 2 to 4 L, but because excess fluid volume is removed by dialysis, the polyuria is not evident. Phases of acute tubular necrosis include:

- Onset (hours to days): GFR decreases in response to ischemia.
- Oliguric/Anuric (5 to 8 days if non-oliguric and 10 to 16 if oliguric): GFR decreases and azotemia occurs.
- Diuretic (7 to 14 days): Kidneys clear fluid but not solutes because of scarring and edema of tubules.
- Recovery: GFR slowly recovers.

96. D: For a hemodialysis cannulation with a blood flow rate of less than 300 mL/min, the needle gauge size that is usually recommended is 17. The faster the blood flow rate, the larger the needle size (and lower the gauge). For blood flow rates of 300 to 350 mL/min, a 16-gauge needle is recommended. If the blood flow rate increases to 350 to 450 mL/min, a 15-gauge needle is recommended and for blood flow rates of more than 450 mL/min, a 14-gauge needle.

97. C: If a dialysis center is utilizing Continuous Quality Improvement methods, the question that the nurse should continually ask is, "How can the center do things better?" The emphasis with CQI is more on process and improving processes to improve efficiency rather than on individuals. CQI focuses on both the needs of internal customers (such as staff) and external customers (such as patients) and is data-driven. CQI also stresses the point that improvement can occur with small steps and should be the concern of all staff rather than just administration.

98. A: The first step in the CQI process is to identify the need for improvement, and this could be a major or minor problem. Once this is identified, then the process must be analyzed through the work of a team that reviews data, studies the problems, and identifies patterns or trends. This usually entails conducting a root cause analysis to determine where the process has failed. The last step is to carry out the plan-do-check-act (PDCA) cycle.

99. C: Early symptoms of disequilibrium syndrome associated with long-term hemodialysis include headache, nausea, and vomiting. While the cause is not clear, it may be due to increased cerebral edema. Acutely uremic patients undergoing hemodialysis may exhibit more severe symptoms, including seizures and coma. Mild cases may be treated symptomatically, but if patients are acutely uremic, the blood flow rate may need to be slowed or dialysis discontinued.

100. D: If an 80-year-old patient with ESKD is a candidate for hemodialysis, but the patient refuses treatment, the nurse should respect the patient's decision, recognizing that patients have a legal and moral right to self-determination. The Patient Self-Determination Act specifically gives people the right to refuse treatment and requires that hospitals and other healthcare facilities and organizations provide information about advance directives to ensure patients' wishes are respected.

101. C: If a patient with diabetes mellitus at high risk for kidney disease shows negative for macroscopic protein with dipstick testing, the nurse expects the next step to be testing for microalbuminuria because early diagnosis is essential to prevent further deterioration of function. Serum creatinine may remain normal until the GRF has fallen to less than 60 mL/min/1.73 m². Normal albumin excretion is 2 to 30 mg/day while microalbuminuria is 30 to 300 mg/day and macroalbuminuria is greater than 300 mg/day.

102. A: All hemodialysis patients should be screened for insomnia because up to 50% of patients have some degree of insomnia, which can adversely affect their quality of life and their abilities to interact socially and carry out activities of daily living. Patients are at increased risk of accidents, and many experience increased depression because of the lack of adequate sleep. The causes of insomnia may be physical or psychosocial, or some combination. Dialysis patients are also at increased risk of other sleep disorders, such as restless legs syndrome, obstructive sleep apnea, and periodic limb movements in sleep.

103. B: The most important factor in preventing exsanguination from dialysis line separation is access site visibility. Because the blood is pumped through the system at the rate of 350 to 500 mL/min, the patient can lose total volume of blood within 10 minutes. While patient education is important, patients often fall asleep during treatment. Venous needle dislodgment is not always detected by alarms, so alarms should not be solely relied on. HemaClips are important safety additions, but should not replace observation.

104. A: If a sentinel event occurs, such as a death resulting from exsanguination, the initial response must include conducting a root cause analysis to determine where the processes failed and whether standards of care were met. Root cause analysis is done retrospectively to determine causes and may involve review of records, interviews, and observations. The focus should be on identifying the process that failed rather than assigning blame. A review of literature should also be included to review current best practices.

105. C: The pH of dialysate usually ranges from 7 to 7.4, which is close to the pH of blood, which usually ranges from 7.35 to 7.45, making it a weak base. It is important for the dialysate to be near the pH of blood so that the pH of the blood does not change during the dialysis process. A solution is acidic if the pH is less than 7 and alkaline if the pH is greater than 7. A pH of 7 is neutral. Some equipment monitors pH throughout dialysis, but pH must always be checked to ensure it is at a safe level.

106. D: If patient on hemodialysis has a myocardial infarction and remains weak but has not resumed any exercise because of fear of another MI, she may benefit the most from a referral to cardiac rehabilitation program. Cardiac rehabilitation programs often offer support services, such as counseling and peer groups, as well as physical recovery services, such as physical and/or occupational therapy, tailored to the patient's abilities and needs. Patients may feel more secure in a sheltered environment when beginning an exercise program.

107. D: The agency that sets the minimally adequate target spKt/V (currently 1.4) as a clinical performance measure for all out-patient dialysis centers in the United States is the Centers for Medicare and Medicaid Services (CMS), based on the guidelines established by National Kidney Foundation Kidney Disease Outcomes Quality Initiative (NKF KDOQI). CMS was required by the Balanced Budget Act to establish measures to determine the quality of renal dialysis services paid for my Medicare/Medicaid.

108. C: If the electronic event-reporting documentation form for the dialysis center is lengthy and time-consuming and not always applicable to the dialysis unit, the best solution is to identify those elements of the form that need modification. Electronic records can usually be modified to some extent to meet the needs of different departments, so the staff should meet with computer technologists who manage the electronic records.

109. A: If a patient has pain and tightness in the chest with pain radiating to the jaw and down the left arm, the nurse's immediate intervention should be to slow the blood flow rate to 150 mL/min as this decreases the amount of stress on the heart. The ultrafiltration rate should also be decreased to slow loss of fluid as this may further stress the heart. The patient's vital signs should be assessed and the physician notified. If the patient is hypotensive, a bolus of saline is indicated. Oxygen may be administered if the patient is dyspneic.

110. C: The potassium level in dialysate is commonly 2.0 mM. If the patient's potassium level is <4.5 mEq/L, then the potassium level of the dialysate may be increased to 3 mM. Patients may require sodium polystyrene sulfonate resin (Kayexalate) to prevent hyperkalemia during treatment. Dialysate with 1 mM potassium should be used only for very short periods because this level has been associated with increased risk of cardiac arrest.

111. C: If a new dialyzer is to be reused, it must be reprocessed and tested to determine the baseline total cell volume (TCV) (or fiber bundle volume), which is the total volume of blood that the blood compartment of this particular dialyzer can hold. In order to be used again, the dialyzer must be checked again to ensure that the TCV for this dialyzer is at least 80% of baseline. The dialyzer cannot be reused if the TCV is lower than 80% because the 20% drop in TCV will result in a 10% decrease in clearance of urea.

112. D: A normal adult man makes about 180 L of glomerular filtrate every 24 hours (or about 125 mL every minute). Glomerular filtrate is the fluid and solutes (such as glucose, amino acids, creatinine, urea, and ions) that are removed from the blood and filtered into Bowman's capsule as the blood is pumped through the glomerulus. Large cells, such as proteins, usually do not filter out of the blood unless there is damage to the nephron. Most of the filtrate is reabsorbed back into the blood in the tubules.

113. A: The 2 hormones secreted by the kidneys are erythropoietin and calcitriol. Erythropoietin stimulates the bone marrow to increase production of red blood cells. Without adequate erythropoietin, the patient develops anemia; therefore, an erythropoiesis-stimulating agent (ESA) may be ordered to increase red blood cell production. Calcitriol is derived from calciferol, which is synthesized by the skin after exposure to ultraviolet light or ingested in the diet (as from vitamin D–enriched dairy products). The liver converts calciferol to vitamin D3, which is converted to calcitriol by the kidneys. Calcitriol promotes absorption of calcium and phosphate.

114. C: The number 1 cause of kidney failure in the United States is type 2 diabetes mellitus, accounting for about 40% of the overall cases. Type 1 diabetes (which is less common) results in about 4% of the total. Because some ethnic groups, such as African Americans, Native Americans, and Hispanics, have high rates of diabetes, they are also at increased risk of kidney failure. Diabetes causes cardiovascular changes, and the changes in the small vessels in the kidney impair the kidney's ability to function.

115. B: Nighttime hemodialysis with 7- to 8-hour sessions 3 times weekly has a number of advantages, including a better survival rate, because patients have about twice as many hours of dialysis compared with the usual daytime schedule (3 times a week for 3 to 4 hours). Patients also have fewer food and fluid restrictions. Patients have fewer complications because the slower hemodialysis is less damaging to the cardiovascular system and removes more of the β-2 M protein that causes amyloidosis.

Section Description: Washington Case Questions

116. C: If a hospitalized patient is newly diagnosed with kidney failure and in need of peritoneal dialysis, but he has little income, inadequate insurance, and little social support, the best initial referral is to a social worker that can assess the patient's resources and needs. The social worker can advise the patient about eligibility for Medicaid and other services in the community and make appropriate referrals to enable the patient to manage the condition.

117. D: When instructing a patient in the use of a preattached double bag system for peritoneal dialysis, the patient should be advised to flush 100 mL of dialysate from the fill bag to the drainage bag before filling the peritoneal cavity. This procedure removes residual air from the tubing. The fill bag (afferent limb of the Y) is opened by breaking a frangible device in the tubing. After flushing, the efferent limb is clamped and the afferent limb unclamped.

118. A: The primary advantage of a 2-compartment peritoneal dialysis solution bag is to allow delivery at normal pH. Standard lactate-based dialysate has a pH of 5.5 because heat sterilization of glucose generates fewer glucose degradation products at low pH; however, low pH may also cause pain during inflow. Additionally, low pH may impair both the immune response to bacteria and the peritoneal membrane, so with 2-compartment dialysate, the smaller portion that contains glucose is heated at a very low pH and the other portion at a higher pH and then the fluids are mixed before administration to achieve normal pH.

119. C: The 3 transport processes that occur at the same time during the course of peritoneal dialysis are as follows:

23. Diffusion: solutes move from the dialysate into the capillary blood and from the capillary blood into the dialysate, depending on various factors, including the concentration gradient and molecular weight of solutes
24. Ultrafiltration: occurs because of the presence of an osmotic agent, such as glucose
25. Absorption: fluid is absorbed via lymphatics and the parietal peritoneum

Section Description: Garcia Case Questions

120. B: If a patient is receiving hemodialysis with a 17-gauge needle but has a blood flow rate of 450 mL/min, the needle is too small for the flow rate, and this can result in hemolysis, which is characterized by hypertension, chest tightness, back pain, and dyspnea, as well as reddening skin color and port-wine appearing blood in the venous line. If a blood sample is centrifuged, the plasma may be pink-tinged because of the breakdown of red blood cells.

121. C: Based on the patient's symptoms, the immediate action should be to stop the blood pump and clamp the blood lines. The hemolyzed blood should be discarded and not reinfused back into the patient. The hemolysis may continue even after dialysis is discontinued, so the patient must be monitored very carefully. The hematocrit may show a marked decrease if hemolysis is extensive. Hemolysis may also occur if there is obstruction or kinking of the arterial blood line.

122. A: The patient should be carefully monitored for hyperkalemia because the hemolysis releases potassium from the red blood cells, and the serum potassium level may increase, putting the patient at risk for muscle weakness and ECG abnormalities that can lead to cardiac arrest. The patient may require additional dialysis or sodium/potassium ion exchange resin orally or rectally to decrease potassium level. Potassium levels:

- Normal values: 3.5 to 5.5 mEq/L
- Hypokalemia: <3.5 mEq/L; Critical value: <2.5 mEq/L
- Hyperkalemia: >5.5 mEq/L; Critical value: >6.5 mEq/L

123. C: According to KDOQI guidelines, patients receiving hemodialysis (or peritoneal dialysis) should receive treatment with an active vitamin D sterol (such as calcitriol) when parathyroid hormone (PTH) levels are greater than 300 pg/mL. Calcitriol is usually administered IV because oral calcitriol is less effective. Normal PTH values are 150 to 300 pg/mL. During treatment with an active vitamin D sterol, levels of calcium, phosphorus, and serum PTH must be monitored and managed separately, depending on values.

124. C: The statement by a patient on hemodialysis that most suggests that the patient may need a referral for psychological counseling is: "Some days I wish I didn't even wake up." Discontent with hemodialysis is common, and expressing those feelings can be helpful for patients. However, many patients become less adherent over time, and many develop depression. Therefore, it is important to listen carefully for indications of depression or suicidal ideation and to actively question the patient about thoughts of suicide.

125. B: If a patient on hemodialysis persists in smoking despite attempts to educate about the risks of smoking, the nurse should advise the patient that nicotine levels after smoking are higher in dialysis patients than in people without kidney disease. Thus, the patient may experience more adverse effects than his parents or siblings, who also smoke but do not have kidney disease. Smoking increases the risk of cardiovascular disease, which is the primary cause of death among patients undergoing dialysis.

Section Description: Independent Questions, Group 3

126. A: The amount of dialysis that a hemodialysis patient is prescribed is based on the removal of urea. Both the removal of urea and the serum level should be monitored, but the removal level is more important than the serum level. Serum levels may at times be within normal range even though removal is inadequate (and vice versa) because the rate of urea generation varies from patient to patient depending on many factors, including nutritional status.

127. D: The use of topical anesthetics, such as EMLA, to reduce discomfort during cannulation is contraindicated for buttonhole sites because the topical anesthetics should be used only on intact skin. Even when used on intact skin, the topical anesthetic should be used only for 1 to 2 weeks and not for long-term cannulation. EMLA is usually applied to the skin and covered with an airtight dressing or plastic wrap and left in place for at least an hour before needle sticks.

128. A: There are 3 different tests associated with hepatitis B:

- Hepatitis B core antibody (HBcAb): A positive finding means the patient has been exposed to the hepatitis B virus.
- Hepatitis B surface antibody (HBsAb): A negative finding means that the patient has never been exposed. A positive finding occurs if the patient has had a previous infection or immunization that has conferred immunity.
- Hepatitis B surface antigen (HbsAg): A positive finding means the patient is infected and can spread the disease.

129. D: As chronic kidney disease progresses from stage 2 to stage 3, the focus of clinical intervention moves toward evaluating and treating complications. The plans for the 5 stages of chronic kidney disease are as follows:

26. Diagnosing and establishing treatment plan as well as reducing risk of cardiovascular disease and slowing disease progression.
27. Monitoring the progression of the disease.
28. Evaluating and treating complications, as kidney function is increasingly impaired.
29. Preparing the patient for eventual dialysis and/or kidney transplant so that patient understands requirements and options.
30. Educating and assisting patient to undergo dialysis and, if appropriate, prepare for transplantation.

130. A: Healthcare personnel caring for patients undergoing kidney transplantation should receive an annual influenza immunization. The CDC recommendations for healthcare personnel also include the hepatitis B series, varicella, and measles, mumps, and rubella (MMR) if not already immune, and a single dose of Tdap. Once an adult has received the Tdap vaccination, subsequent boosters should be with Td every 10 years. Family members and caregivers should also be advised to have the same immunizations in order to protect the patient.

131. D: If a patient with a donor kidney develops sudden onset of hypertension 2 years after transplantation, the most likely cause is arterial stenosis, which can occur in up to 10% of patients within a few months or years after transplantation. Angiography is usually done to exclude other diagnoses and confirm stenosis. Treatment most commonly involves angioplasty and stent placement in order to ensure patency of the artery. Doppler ultrasonography may be used postoperatively to monitor progress and assess for hematoma formation.

132. A: If, following kidney transplantation, a patient develops a large lymphocele between the bladder and the transplanted kidney, the treatment of choice is usually internal drainage into the abdomen, done laparoscopically. A lymphocele usually develops within the first year when lymphatic vessels leak lymph into the tissues. Patients typically complain of edema and pain and exhibit impairment of renal function. If the lymphocele is very small, sclerotherapy may be used, but the lymphocele may recur. Aspiration may increase risk of infection, especially if a drainage catheter is left in place. Fibrin glue is sometimes used.

133. B: Amino acid–based solution for peritoneal dialysis is indicated for nutritionally compromised patients and is essentially absorbed by the end of a 4- to 6-hour dwell. Amino acid–based solutions can only be used once per day because more frequent use may result in acidosis and increased blood urea. Amino acid–based solution is more effective with oral intake of adequate calories, which is needed for protein synthesis. If a patient has poor intake of food, then the amino acid–based solution may be administered with glucose.

134. C: An upper chest presternal exit site for peritoneal dialysis may be indicated for patients who are morbidly obese. Presternal exit sites may also be used in patients who have an existing stoma as well as those who have a history of tunnel infection and those who are incontinent and wear adult diapers, resulting in increased risk of infection. Some advantages include the ability to take a tub bath and decreased irritation from clothing. The site also has less movement, so the catheter is more stable.

135. D: Mixing aminoglycosides (such as gentamicin, amikacin, netilmicin, paromomycin, and tobramycin) in the same dialysis solution bag with penicillins (a beta-lactam) is contraindicated because the drugs are incompatible. The penicillin may react with the aminoglycoside and interfere with the action of the aminoglycoside, rendering it less effective. Additionally, kidney disease may exacerbate this reaction. Antibiotics that can be mixed with penicillins include vancomycin and cephalosporins, such as cefazolin and ceftazidime.

136. D: Vancomycin is stable in dialysate stored at room temperature for up to 28 days, but high ambient temperatures may render the antibiotic unstable earlier. Gentamicin (an aminoglycoside) is stable at room temperature for 14 days; if the solution contains heparin, this reduces the duration. Cefazolin (a cephalosporin) is stable at room temperature for 8 days and under refrigeration for 14 days, while ceftazidime (another cephalosporin) is stable for only 4 days at room temperature and 7 days if refrigerated.

137. B: If a patient on peritoneal dialysis tells the nurse that one of the employees at his company has offered to give him a kidney in exchange for $100,000, the nurse should advise the patient that it is illegal to buy or sell an organ. The patient could encounter both criminal and civil penalties, especially if the employee later claims coercion or suffers adverse effects. Additionally, the patient may be subjected to blackmail because of the illegal nature of the transaction.

138. A: If a female patient with CAPD has become increasingly withdrawn and is reluctant to be seen in public unless wearing a large coat, the patient is most likely experiencing body image disturbance. This is common because of abdominal distention and weight gain associated with CAPD. Additionally, lifestyle changes that are required to accommodate CAPD can challenge a patient's perception of self. Some patients may benefit from a fashion consultation to help them to pick appropriate clothing that is stylish and flattering.

139. D: Considering the peritoneal equilibrium test (PET), patients categorized as high transporters would be expected to have the highest 4-hour dialysate to plasma creatinine, urea, and sodium (D/PCr, PUr, and PNa) values, usually because of a large and effective peritoneal surface area and/or highly permeable membrane. However, dialysate glucose also diffuses quickly into the blood for the same reasons, resulting in low 4-hour dialysate to dialysate zero glucose values (D/D_0G). High transporters also tend to have higher loss of protein and serum albumin.

140. D: Potassium and uremic solutes diffuse from peritoneal capillary blood into peritoneal fluid during peritoneal dialysis while glucose and lactate or bicarbonate as well as calcium and magnesium diffuse in the opposite direction, from the dialysate into the capillary blood. Some potassium is also released from the peritoneal lining during dialysis. Potassium is commonly added to dialysate to compensate for the loss that occurs during treatment. Patients should be advised to eat foods high in potassium (3000 to 4000 mg/day is recommended).

141. A: If a patient with CAPD has decreased effluent volumes of dialysate and increased weight gain without peripheral edema, and physical examination shows an asymmetric protuberant abdomen, the most likely cause is abdominal wall leak. The weight gain occurs as the fluid builds up in the abdominal wall tissues. The patient should stand during examination of the abdomen as asymmetry is more readily identified in this position. Abdominal wall leaks may result from poor surgical technique. The patient may need to convert to day dry APD or hemodialysis until the defect in the wall heals.

142. A: If an infection occurs in an arteriovenous graft, the patient is at increased risk of hemorrhage because the infection may cause the graft material to disintegrate. Grafts may be biologic, semi-biologic, or prosthetic (most commonly made from Teflon or fabric) and are implanted to form an anastomosis between a vein and artery. Arteriovenous grafts pose a greater risk of infection than arteriovenous fistulas and have a shorter life span, typically 2 to 3 years.

143. B: If a patient has active infectious tuberculosis and has been receiving hemodialysis, the treatments should be continued in an isolation room with negative airflow, usually in an acute care facility. In some cases, this may mean that the patient must receive treatment in a different facility if a negative airflow room is not available. As a precaution, hemodialysis patients and staff should be required to have yearly TB skin tests and to take medications to treat or prevent infections as indicated.

144. A: If a dialysis patient presents with shaking chills, high fever, myalgia, hypotension, nausea, and vomiting, the most likely causative agents are gram-negative bacteria. Sources of possible contamination include the water processing system, hemodialyzer reprocessing/priming, and ultrafilter waste disposal. Internal sources of gram-negative bacteria, such as perforation of the bowel, should be eliminated. Less commonly, endotoxins may cause a similar reaction with hypotension, fever, and chills, and may progress to multiple organ failure.

Section Description: Lee Case Questions

145. D: The purpose of "vessel mapping" is to ensure that the physician will find adequate vessels for the AV fistula. Vessel mapping uses Doppler ultrasound to assess vessels. The normal rate of blood flow in the brachial artery in a patient with ESKD is less than 100 mL/min, but the AV fistula must be able to accommodate much higher volumes (up to 1200 mL/min for radiocephalic fistula and up to 1500 mL/min for brachiocephalic fistula), so choosing a vessel that can dilate sufficiently is critical.

146. C: During the first week of treatment with a new AV fistula, the initial flow rate is kept at 200 to 250 mL/min. The physician will determine when the flow rate should increase, based on feedback provided by cannulators. New AV fistula should never be cannulated by inexperienced staff.

147. A: When determining if a new AV fistula is maturing, the 3 factors to assess by palpation are the thrill, vessel growth, and vessel firmness. The thrill should not have the character of a pulse but should be a constant vibratory sensation. The vessel should begin to grow soon after surgery and should be evident by 2 weeks. The growth should be assessed for evenness and any flat spots, which may indicate stenosis, noted. The vessel should become firmer as the vessel becomes stronger.

148. D: If a patient is referred to physical therapy for exercises to mature a fistula that was created 1 week earlier in the lower arm, the exercises likely include ball squeeze to slow blood return and dilate the fistula. Other exercises include squeezing and opening a clothespin for 5 minutes or touching fingers to thumb tip. Exercises are done for 5 to 10 minutes up to 6 times daily. Exercises for fistulas in the upper arm include hammer and bicep curls using light weights, 1 to 3 pounds.

149. C: During the first week of treatment with a new AV fistula, the initial needle size is usually #17 gauge because a larger needle may damage the fistula, especially if it infiltrates. The initial flow rate is also kept low at 200 to 250 mL/min.

150. B: With an AV fistula, cannulation should be done at an angle of 25° to 35°. Improperly cannulating an AV fistula may result in pain and anxiety on the part of the patient and premature failure of the access site. AV grafts should be cannulated at an angle of about 45°. Steps to cannulation include inspecting the AV site and arm for discoloration or breaks in the skin, palpating for a thrill, and auscultating to assess the flow of blood and the bruit.

151. D: According to the "Rule of 6s," an AV fistula is considered successful it if is 0.6 cm wide, is positioned less than 0.6 cm below the skin surface, and has a blood flow rate of at least 600 mL/min as verified by ultrasound. The AV fistula is the recommended access for hemodialysis because it is the longest lasting and tends to have a lower risk of blood clotting. Use of the patient's own vessels is preferred. One problem with the AV fistula is that it can take 1 to 4 months to mature, during which an alternate access is required.

152. A: According to the KDOQI, the minimum hemodialysis session length for a patient with little residual urine volume is 3 hours, 3 times a week. In the United States, sessions lasting 3.5 to 4 hours, 3 times per week are common for patients treated in dialysis centers. Patients on home dialysis often do more frequent treatments, such as 5 to 7 days a week. Some patients routinely do nighttime hemodialysis with some dialysis centers offering in-center overnight treatment with sessions lasting from 6 to 9 hours.

153. D: If after initiation of calcitriol treatment for elevated PTH level the patient's calcium level is 10.5 mg/dL, the appropriate response is to hold the calcitriol, because the level is greater than 10.2 mg/dL. High levels of calcium are associated with vascular calcification and increased mortality rates, especially if levels are greater than 12 mg/dL. Levels lower than 7 mg/dL also increase risks. The optimal level for patients is 9 to 12 mg/dL, but giving calcitriol at levels greater than 10.2 mg/dL may cause the level to increase over 12 mg/dL.

Section Description: Yager Case Questions

154. B: After implantation of a prosthetic arteriovenous graft, maturation usually takes 3 to 6 weeks; some graft material can be used as soon as the graft has healed, after about 2 weeks. The AV graft is usually done when a patient lacks adequate vessels for formation of an AV fistula. The AV graft is easier to access than an AV fistula but has a shorter life expectancy and is more prone to complications. The graft may be straight or looped.

155. B: If routine heparin (unfractionated) is administered for anticoagulation for hemodialysis with an initial bolus (usually 2000 units) and subsequent infusion, the correct administration is to inject the bolus into the venous line, flush with saline, and then infuse heparin (usually 1200 units per hour) into the arterial line. An alternative method for routine heparinization is to administer an initial higher bolus (such as 4000 units) and then give 1000 to 2000 unit boluses as need.

156. C: After the initial heparin bolus for hemodialysis, dialysis should be initiated in 3 to 5 minutes, which provides times for the heparin to disperse. Anticoagulation is important during dialysis because the blood must come in contact with a variety of different surfaces and membranes, all of which may result in the thrombus formation and blood clotting. Without anticoagulation, the thrombus formation may result in occlusion within the circuit.

157. D: Heparin should generally be administered during hemodialysis to maintain an ACT level of baseline plus 80%. The level at the end of dialysis should be baseline plus 40%. If patients are at risk for bleeding and heparin-free dialysis resulted in clotting, then a tight heparin protocol is followed. With tight heparin, the ACT should be maintained at baseline plus 40% during dialysis and at the end of dialysis. The initial bolus dose is lower, 750 units, and the heparin infusion is initiated at the rate of 600 units per hour, but adjusted to maintain baseline plus 40%.

158. A: When teaching a patient on hemodialysis to intake, the nurse advises the patient that fluid intake should be based on 1000 mL/day (this may vary according to individuals) plus the amount of urine in the preceding 24-hour period, in this case 500 mL. Thus, the patient is allowed 1500 mL/day intake. As the time lengthens between treatments, fluid retention usually increases and urinary output decreases, so fluid intake is increasingly restricted.

159. D: If 5 minutes after initiation of a hemodialysis treatment the patient complains of dyspnea, generalized edema, tingling about the mouth, and feeling faint, and has periorbital edema and hives, the nurse should immediately call for help and clamp all lines and stop the hemodialysis. Because these symptoms are consistent with anaphylaxis, blood in the system should not be returned to the patient as this may increase the allergic response. Oxygen may be administered to relieve dyspnea. Epinephrine may be administered to control anaphylaxis.

Section Description: Mayer Case Questions

160. B: If a patient with symptoms of acute glomerulonephritis also presents with malar rash, arthralgias, and oral lesions, these findings are suggestive of systemic lupus erythematosus (SLE), which is a common noninfectious cause of acute glomerulonephritis. SLE is a multi-system autoimmune disorder. With SLE, the injury to the glomeruli is related to deposition of immune complexes. Lupus nephritis commonly occurs within 5 years of diagnosis of SLE as the disease progresses. The patient is also at increased risk of cardiovascular disease.

161. D: Based on these findings, the patient may require consultation with a rheumatologist because the treatment approach is different from that utilized with infectious causes of acute glomerulonephritis. For example, steroids may be indicated for SLE and are contraindicated for infectious glomerulonephritis. Symptoms associated with SLE may be varied, and treatment challenging, so a physician with expertise in treating SLE should be consulted prior to beginning treatment if possible.

Section Description: Infection Case Questions

162. C: The greatest risk of bacteremia occurs with dialysis catheters with the overall infection risk 7 times greater than for patients with an arteriovenous fistula. If a patient is not a candidate for an AV fistula, then an AV graft should be the next choice. Dialysis catheters should be used only for acute dialysis with an expected duration of less than 3 weeks; if a longer time is required, then the catheter should be tunneled and cuffed with insertion in the right internal jugular vein.

163. B: The 3 blood borne pathogens that pose the most risk for hemodialysis patients are hepatitis B, hepatitis C, and HIV. Hepatitis B is highly contagious and may be spread from contaminated vials, surfaces, and drugs, as well as from individuals who are infected. Patients should be advised to have the hepatitis B vaccination to protect them from infection. Hepatitis C spreads less readily than hepatitis B but still poses risk. HIV is also spread through blood and body fluids.

164. A: According to the NQF criteria, when calculating the Standardized Infection Ratio (SIR) of bloodstream infections (BSIs) for patients treated in an ambulatory hemodialysis center, the data that would be used for the numerator is the number of positive blood cultures drawn from outpatients of an ambulatory hemodialysis center or within 1 day of their hospitalization. The denominator data would be the number of patients treated in the ambulatory hemodialysis center on the first 2 working days of the month.

165. C: Chlorhexidine gluconate 2% is the antiseptic with the broadest spectrum antibacterial activity used for skin prep for a fistula site, and this solution is recommended by the CDC. The solution should be applied back and forth (not in a circle) to the site for 30 seconds, as this is the time needed for activation. Antisepsis persists for up to 48 hours after cleansing. The solution should air dry. In some cases, chlorhexidine gluconate 2% is combined with isopropyl alcohol 70%. If used alone, alcohol must be applied for 1 minute and povidone iodine for 2 to 3 minutes.

166. D: The purpose of a break tank or reduced pressure zone valve in the water system is to prevent backflow. If water pressure falls in the water distribution system, such as may occur with a line break or high water demand, water connected to the supply line from underground sources or storage tanks may backflow into the water system, resulting in contaminations. The break tank or reduced pressure zone valve prevents chemicals that have been removed during dialysis from entering the public water system and prevents contaminated water from entering the water distribution system.

167. C: While a patient is undergoing hemodialysis, chloramine testing should be conducted every 4 hours. Carbon filters are used to remove chloramine, chorine, and organic material from public water supplies. If the chloramine is not removed, it can result in red blood cell hemolysis. The carbon filters may become contaminated with bacteria. Water should be warmed and at least 2 carbon filters used in a series. Prior to testing, the system should be functioning for at least 15 minutes with testing done after the first carbon tank.

168. A: The last component of the water processing system before the distribution loop should be an ultrafilter, which is used with or without ultraviolet lights to remove bacteria and endotoxins from the water supply used for dialysis. In some cases, an ultrafilter may also be placed before the reverse osmosis. Even with the ultrafilters in place, the water supply must be monitored for bacteria and endotoxins because ultrafilters do not remove 100% of all contaminants.

169. B: Fluoride contamination of water used for hemodialysis may result in ventricular fibrillation, which can lead to cardiac arrest. Other symptoms of excessive fluoride include bone disease, pruritus, nausea and vomiting, and chest pain. Fluoride contamination results from inadequate treatment of water. The acceptable level of fluoride is 0.2 ppm, but the level can increase, for example, if a deionizer is exhausted. A deionizer should have both audio and visual alarms, and all staff should be trained to understand the monitoring system in use.

170. D: Aluminum, which is a contaminant that can be found in water used for dialysis, may result in dialysis dementia. Aluminum toxicity may occur with chronic kidney disease and in patients receiving aluminum-containing dialysate (associated with the aluminum content of the water) and taking aluminum salts as treatment of hyperphosphatemia. Patients may develop encephalopathy, first characterized by difficulties with speech and then dementia, seizures, and myoclonus. Excess aluminum may also cause anemia, osteomalacia, and osteodystrophy.

171. C: The external surface of the hemodialysis machine should be cleansed and disinfected after every patient. If water or dialysate has sat in the hemodialysis machine overnight, then all of the fluid distribution system must be disinfected prior to the first utilization of the equipment for hemodialysis in the morning. Care must be taken to ensure that waste does not backflow into the machine. Most hemodialysis machines in the United States are single-pass machines in which all dialysate is discarded through a drain.

172. B: In order for the reverse osmosis (RO) equipment that is part of the water treatment system to work properly, the water temperature must be maintained at 77 °F to 82 °F (25 °C to 28 °C). As the water enters the system, hot and cold water is mixed to the correct temperature by a temperature-blending valve and verified by an inline thermometer. If the water temperature falls below this level by 1 °C, the product flow decreases by 3% and solute removal increases. Temperatures in excess of 95 °F (35 °C) may damage the reverse osmosis membrane.

Section Description: Walker Case Questions

173. B: Nonadherence to treatment plans is quite common in patients with kidney failure, especially younger patients or those with limited social support, because of the limitations treatment poses. The best approach is to avoid criticizing or giving advice but to ask the patient how the nurse can help her better manage her condition. This approach shows respect for the patient as an adult who is free to make her own decisions about treatment and engages her in a cooperative process of change.

174. B: Adult polycystic kidney disease (PKD) is an autosomal dominant disorder, so a patient of childbearing age with this disease may be referred to a genetics counselor when considering pregnancy because the disease may be passed on to children. Pregnant patients are also at increased risk of preeclampsia. PKD causes cysts to form in the kidneys and sometimes other organs, such as the liver.

Patients often develop hypertension, chronic pain, mitral valve prolapse, and diverticulosis, and some progress to kidney failure.

175. A: If a nurse feels a special friendship toward a kidney failure patient who reminds the nurse of a close family member, the nurse should deal with this by acknowledging the feeling. It is not unusual to feel more positively or more negatively toward some patients than others, but the important factor is the ability to recognize these biases and to act in a professional manner, providing the same level of attention and care to all patients.

How to Overcome Test Anxiety

Just the thought of taking a test is enough to make most people a little nervous. A test is an important event that can have a long-term impact on your future, so it's important to take it seriously and it's natural to feel anxious about performing well. But just because anxiety is normal, that doesn't mean that it's helpful in test taking, or that you should simply accept it as part of your life. Anxiety can have a variety of effects. These effects can be mild, like making you feel slightly nervous, or severe, like blocking your ability to focus or remember even a simple detail.

If you experience test anxiety—whether severe or mild—it's important to know how to beat it. To discover this, first you need to understand what causes test anxiety.

Causes of Test Anxiety

While we often think of anxiety as an uncontrollable emotional state, it can actually be caused by simple, practical things. One of the most common causes of test anxiety is that a person does not feel adequately prepared for their test. This feeling can be the result of many different issues such as poor study habits or lack of organization, but the most common culprit is time management. Starting to study too late, failing to organize your study time to cover all of the material, or being distracted while you study will mean that you're not well prepared for the test. This may lead to cramming the night before, which will cause you to be physically and mentally exhausted for the test. Poor time management also contributes to feelings of stress, fear, and hopelessness as you realize you are not well prepared but don't know what to do about it.

Other times, test anxiety is not related to your preparation for the test but comes from unresolved fear. This may be a past failure on a test, or poor performance on tests in general. It may come from comparing yourself to others who seem to be performing better or from the stress of living up to expectations. Anxiety may be driven by fears of the future—how failure on this test would affect your educational and career goals. These fears are often completely irrational, but they can still negatively impact your test performance.

> **Review Video: 3 Reasons You Have Test Anxiety**
> Visit mometrix.com/academy and enter code: 428468

Elements of Test Anxiety

As mentioned earlier, test anxiety is considered to be an emotional state, but it has physical and mental components as well. Sometimes you may not even realize that you are suffering from test anxiety until you notice the physical symptoms. These can include trembling hands, rapid heartbeat, sweating, nausea, and tense muscles. Extreme anxiety may lead to fainting or vomiting. Obviously, any of these symptoms can have a negative impact on testing. It is important to recognize them as soon as they begin to occur so that you can address the problem before it damages your performance.

> **Review Video: 3 Ways to Tell You Have Test Anxiety**
> Visit mometrix.com/academy and enter code: 927847

The mental components of test anxiety include trouble focusing and inability to remember learned information. During a test, your mind is on high alert, which can help you recall information and stay focused for an extended period of time. However, anxiety interferes with your mind's natural processes, causing you to blank out, even on the questions you know well. The strain of testing during anxiety makes it difficult to stay focused, especially on a test that may take several hours. Extreme anxiety can take a huge mental toll, making it difficult not only to recall test information but even to understand the test questions or pull your thoughts together.

> **Review Video: How Test Anxiety Affects Memory**
> Visit mometrix.com/academy and enter code: 609003

Effects of Test Anxiety

Test anxiety is like a disease—if left untreated, it will get progressively worse. Anxiety leads to poor performance, and this reinforces the feelings of fear and failure, which in turn lead to poor performances on subsequent tests. It can grow from a mild nervousness to a crippling condition. If allowed to progress, test anxiety can have a big impact on your schooling, and consequently on your future.

Test anxiety can spread to other parts of your life. Anxiety on tests can become anxiety in any stressful situation, and blanking on a test can turn into panicking in a job situation. But fortunately, you don't have to let anxiety rule your testing and determine your grades. There are a number of relatively simple steps you can take to move past anxiety and function normally on a test and in the rest of life.

> **Review Video: How Test Anxiety Impacts Your Grades**
> Visit mometrix.com/academy and enter code: 939819

Physical Steps for Beating Test Anxiety

While test anxiety is a serious problem, the good news is that it can be overcome. It doesn't have to control your ability to think and remember information. While it may take time, you can begin taking steps today to beat anxiety.

Just as your first hint that you may be struggling with anxiety comes from the physical symptoms, the first step to treating it is also physical. Rest is crucial for having a clear, strong mind. If you are tired, it is much easier to give in to anxiety. But if you establish good sleep habits, your body and mind will be ready to perform optimally, without the strain of exhaustion. Additionally, sleeping well helps you to retain information better, so you're more likely to recall the answers when you see the test questions.

Getting good sleep means more than going to bed on time. It's important to allow your brain time to relax. Take study breaks from time to time so it doesn't get overworked, and don't study right before bed. Take time to rest your mind before trying to rest your body, or you may find it difficult to fall asleep.

> **Review Video: The Importance of Sleep for Your Brain**
> Visit mometrix.com/academy and enter code: 319338

Along with sleep, other aspects of physical health are important in preparing for a test. Good nutrition is vital for good brain function. Sugary foods and drinks may give a burst of energy but this burst is followed by a crash, both physically and emotionally. Instead, fuel your body with protein and vitamin-rich foods.

Also, drink plenty of water. Dehydration can lead to headaches and exhaustion, especially if your brain is already under stress from the rigors of the test. Particularly if your test is a long one, drink water during the breaks. And if possible, take an energy-boosting snack to eat between sections.

> **Review Video: How Diet Can Affect your Mood**
> Visit mometrix.com/academy and enter code: 624317

Along with sleep and diet, a third important part of physical health is exercise. Maintaining a steady workout schedule is helpful, but even taking 5-minute study breaks to walk can help get your blood pumping faster and clear your head. Exercise also releases endorphins, which contribute to a positive feeling and can help combat test anxiety.

When you nurture your physical health, you are also contributing to your mental health. If your body is healthy, your mind is much more likely to be healthy as well. So take time to rest, nourish your body with healthy food and water, and get moving as much as possible. Taking these physical steps will make you stronger and more able to take the mental steps necessary to overcome test anxiety.

> **Review Video: How to Stay Healthy and Prevent Test Anxiety**
> Visit mometrix.com/academy and enter code: 877894

Mental Steps for Beating Test Anxiety

Working on the mental side of test anxiety can be more challenging, but as with the physical side, there are clear steps you can take to overcome it. As mentioned earlier, test anxiety often stems from lack of preparation, so the obvious solution is to prepare for the test. Effective studying may be the most important weapon you have for beating test anxiety, but you can and should employ several other mental tools to combat fear.

First, boost your confidence by reminding yourself of past success—tests or projects that you aced. If you're putting as much effort into preparing for this test as you did for those, there's no reason you should expect to fail here. Work hard to prepare; then trust your preparation.

Second, surround yourself with encouraging people. It can be helpful to find a study group, but be sure that the people you're around will encourage a positive attitude. If you spend time with others who are anxious or cynical, this will only contribute to your own anxiety. Look for others who are motivated to study hard from a desire to succeed, not from a fear of failure.

Third, reward yourself. A test is physically and mentally tiring, even without anxiety, and it can be helpful to have something to look forward to. Plan an activity following the test, regardless of the outcome, such as going to a movie or getting ice cream.

When you are taking the test, if you find yourself beginning to feel anxious, remind yourself that you know the material. Visualize successfully completing the test. Then take a few deep, relaxing breaths and return to it. Work through the questions carefully but with confidence, knowing that you are capable of succeeding.

Developing a healthy mental approach to test taking will also aid in other areas of life. Test anxiety affects more than just the actual test—it can be damaging to your mental health and even contribute to depression. It's important to beat test anxiety before it becomes a problem for more than testing.

> **Review Video: Test Anxiety and Depression**
> Visit mometrix.com/academy and enter code: 904704

Study Strategy

Being prepared for the test is necessary to combat anxiety, but what does being prepared look like? You may study for hours on end and still not feel prepared. What you need is a strategy for test prep. The next few pages outline our recommended steps to help you plan out and conquer the challenge of preparation.

STEP 1: SCOPE OUT THE TEST

Learn everything you can about the format (multiple choice, essay, etc.) and what will be on the test. Gather any study materials, course outlines, or sample exams that may be available. Not only will this help you to prepare, but knowing what to expect can help to alleviate test anxiety.

STEP 2: MAP OUT THE MATERIAL

Look through the textbook or study guide and make note of how many chapters or sections it has. Then divide these over the time you have. For example, if a book has 15 chapters and you have five days to study, you need to cover three chapters each day. Even better, if you have the time, leave an extra day at the end for overall review after you have gone through the material in depth.

If time is limited, you may need to prioritize the material. Look through it and make note of which sections you think you already have a good grasp on, and which need review. While you are studying, skim quickly through the familiar sections and take more time on the challenging parts. Write out your plan so you don't get lost as you go. Having a written plan also helps you feel more in control of the study, so anxiety is less likely to arise from feeling overwhelmed at the amount to cover.

STEP 3: GATHER YOUR TOOLS

Decide what study method works best for you. Do you prefer to highlight in the book as you study and then go back over the highlighted portions? Or do you type out notes of the important information? Or is it helpful to make flashcards that you can carry with you? Assemble the pens, index cards, highlighters, post-it notes, and any other materials you may need so you won't be distracted by getting up to find things while you study.

If you're having a hard time retaining the information or organizing your notes, experiment with different methods. For example, try color-coding by subject with colored pens, highlighters, or post-it notes. If you learn better by hearing, try recording yourself reading your notes so you can listen while in the car, working out, or simply sitting at your desk. Ask a friend to quiz you from your flashcards, or try teaching someone the material to solidify it in your mind.

STEP 4: CREATE YOUR ENVIRONMENT

It's important to avoid distractions while you study. This includes both the obvious distractions like visitors and the subtle distractions like an uncomfortable chair (or a too-comfortable couch that makes you want to fall asleep). Set up the best study environment possible: good lighting and a comfortable work area. If background music helps you focus, you may want to turn it on, but otherwise keep the room quiet. If you are using a computer to take notes, be sure you don't have any other windows open, especially applications like social media, games, or anything else that could distract you. Silence your phone and turn off notifications. Be sure to keep water close by so you stay hydrated while you study (but avoid unhealthy drinks and snacks).

Also, take into account the best time of day to study. Are you freshest first thing in the morning? Try to set aside some time then to work through the material. Is your mind clearer in the afternoon or evening? Schedule your study session then. Another method is to study at the same time of day that you will take the test, so that your brain gets used to working on the material at that time and will be ready to focus at test time.

STEP 5: STUDY!

Once you have done all the study preparation, it's time to settle into the actual studying. Sit down, take a few moments to settle your mind so you can focus, and begin to follow your study plan. Don't give in to distractions or let yourself procrastinate. This is your time to prepare so you'll be ready to fearlessly approach the test. Make the most of the time and stay focused.

Of course, you don't want to burn out. If you study too long you may find that you're not retaining the information very well. Take regular study breaks. For example, taking five minutes out of every hour to walk briskly, breathing deeply and swinging your arms, can help your mind stay fresh.

As you get to the end of each chapter or section, it's a good idea to do a quick review. Remind yourself of what you learned and work on any difficult parts. When you feel that you've mastered the material, move on to the next part. At the end of your study session, briefly skim through your notes again.

But while review is helpful, cramming last minute is NOT. If at all possible, work ahead so that you won't need to fit all your study into the last day. Cramming overloads your brain with more information than it can process and retain, and your tired mind may struggle to recall even previously learned information when it is overwhelmed with last-minute study. Also, the urgent nature of cramming and the stress placed on your brain contribute to anxiety. You'll be more likely to go to the test feeling unprepared and having trouble thinking clearly.

So don't cram, and don't stay up late before the test, even just to review your notes at a leisurely pace. Your brain needs rest more than it needs to go over the information again. In fact, plan to finish your studies by noon or early afternoon the day before the test. Give your brain the rest of the day to relax or focus on other things, and get a good night's sleep. Then you will be fresh for the test and better able to recall what you've studied.

STEP 6: TAKE A PRACTICE TEST

Many courses offer sample tests, either online or in the study materials. This is an excellent resource to check whether you have mastered the material, as well as to prepare for the test format and environment.

Check the test format ahead of time: the number of questions, the type (multiple choice, free response, etc.), and the time limit. Then create a plan for working through them. For example, if you have 30 minutes to take a 60-question test, your limit is 30 seconds per question. Spend less time on the questions you know well so that you can take more time on the difficult ones.

If you have time to take several practice tests, take the first one open book, with no time limit. Work through the questions at your own pace and make sure you fully understand them. Gradually work up to taking a test under test conditions: sit at a desk with all study materials put away and set a timer. Pace yourself to make sure you finish the test with time to spare and go back to check your answers if you have time.

After each test, check your answers. On the questions you missed, be sure you understand why you missed them. Did you misread the question (tests can use tricky wording)? Did you forget the information? Or was it something you hadn't learned? Go back and study any shaky areas that the practice tests reveal.

Taking these tests not only helps with your grade, but also aids in combating test anxiety. If you're already used to the test conditions, you're less likely to worry about it, and working through tests until you're scoring well gives you a confidence boost. Go through the practice tests until you feel comfortable, and then you can go into the test knowing that you're ready for it.

Test Tips

On test day, you should be confident, knowing that you've prepared well and are ready to answer the questions. But aside from preparation, there are several test day strategies you can employ to maximize your performance.

First, as stated before, get a good night's sleep the night before the test (and for several nights before that, if possible). Go into the test with a fresh, alert mind rather than staying up late to study.

Try not to change too much about your normal routine on the day of the test. It's important to eat a nutritious breakfast, but if you normally don't eat breakfast at all, consider eating just a protein bar. If you're a coffee drinker, go ahead and have your normal coffee. Just make sure you time it so that the caffeine doesn't wear off right in the middle of your test. Avoid sugary beverages, and drink enough water to stay hydrated but not so much that you need a restroom break 10 minutes into the test. If your test isn't first thing in the morning, consider going for a walk or doing a light workout before the test to get your blood flowing.

Allow yourself enough time to get ready, and leave for the test with plenty of time to spare so you won't have the anxiety of scrambling to arrive in time. Another reason to be early is to select a good seat. It's helpful to sit away from doors and windows, which can be distracting. Find a good seat, get out your supplies, and settle your mind before the test begins.

When the test begins, start by going over the instructions carefully, even if you already know what to expect. Make sure you avoid any careless mistakes by following the directions.

Then begin working through the questions, pacing yourself as you've practiced. If you're not sure on an answer, don't spend too much time on it, and don't let it shake your confidence. Either skip it and come back later, or eliminate as many wrong answers as possible and guess among the remaining ones. Don't dwell on these questions as you continue—put them out of your mind and focus on what lies ahead.

Be sure to read all of the answer choices, even if you're sure the first one is the right answer. Sometimes you'll find a better one if you keep reading. But don't second-guess yourself if you do immediately know the answer. Your gut instinct is usually right. Don't let test anxiety rob you of the information you know.

If you have time at the end of the test (and if the test format allows), go back and review your answers. Be cautious about changing any, since your first instinct tends to be correct, but make sure you didn't misread any of the questions or accidentally mark the wrong answer choice. Look over any you skipped and make an educated guess.

At the end, leave the test feeling confident. You've done your best, so don't waste time worrying about your performance or wishing you could change anything. Instead, celebrate the successful completion of this test. And finally, use this test to learn how to deal with anxiety even better next time.

> **Review Video: 5 Tips to Beat Test Anxiety**
> Visit mometrix.com/academy and enter code: 570656

Important Qualification

Not all anxiety is created equal. If your test anxiety is causing major issues in your life beyond the classroom or testing center, or if you are experiencing troubling physical symptoms related to your anxiety, it may be a sign of a serious physiological or psychological condition. If this sounds like your situation, we strongly encourage you to seek professional help.

Tell Us Your Story

We at Mometrix would like to extend our heartfelt thanks to you for letting us be a part of your journey. It is an honor to serve people from all walks of life, people like you, who are committed to building the best future they can for themselves.

We know that each person's situation is unique. But we also know that, whether you are a young student or a mother of four, you care about working to make your own life and the lives of those around you better.

That's why we want to hear your story.

We want to know why you're taking this test. We want to know about the trials you've gone through to get here. And we want to know about the successes you've experienced after taking and passing your test.

In addition to your story, which can be an inspiration both to us and to others, we value your feedback. We want to know both what you loved about our book and what you think we can improve on.

The team at Mometrix would be absolutely thrilled to hear from you! So please, send us an email at tellusyourstory@mometrix.com or visit us at mometrix.com/tellusyourstory.php and let's stay in touch.

Additional Bonus Material

Due to our efforts to try to keep this book to a manageable length, we've created a link that will give you access to all of your additional bonus material.

> Please visit http://www.mometrix.com/bonus948/cdn to access the information.